Creative

Imagery

in Nursing

Creative Imagery in Nursing

KARILEE HALO SHAMES, PhD, RN
Director
Nurse Empowerment Workshops & Services
P.O. Box 2398
Mill Valley, CA 94942

Clinical Specialist, Psychiatric Nursing

California Coordinator, Director-At-Large—National Leadership Council, American Holistic Nurses Association (AHNA)

Certificate in Holistic Nursing, AHNA

Healing Touch Practitioner (Certified) and Instructor, AHNA

Delmar Publishers

 I(T)P™

An International Thomson Publishing Company

Albany • Bonn • Boston • Cincinnati • Detroit • London
Madrid • Melbourne • Mexico City • New York • Pacific (
Paris • San Francisco • Singapore • Tokyo • Toronto • W

NOTICE TO THE READER

Cover Design: Spiral·Design
Cover Illustration: Kirsten Soderlind

Delmar Staff

Publisher: Diane L. McOscar
Senior Acquisitions Editor: Bill Burgower
Assistant Editor: Debra M. Flis
Editorial Assistant: Chrisoula Baikos
Production Manager: Karen Leet
Project Editors: Danya M. Plotsky/Judith Boyd Nelson
Production Coordinator: Barbara A. Bullock
Art and Design Coordinator: Mary E. Siener

COPYRIGHT © 1996
By Delmar Publishers
a division of International Thomson Publishing Inc.

The ITP logo is a trademark under license.

Printed in the United States of America

For more information, contact:

Delmar Publishers
3 Columbia Circle, Box 15015
Albany, New York 12212-5015

International Thomson Publishing Europe
Berkshire House 168-173
High Holborn
London, WC1V 7AA
England

Thomas Nelson Australia
102 Dodds Street
South Melbourne, 3205
Victoria, Australia

Nelson Canada
1120 Birchmont Road
Scarborough, Ontario
Canada, M1K 5G4

International Thomson Editores
Campos Eliseos 385, Piso 7
Col Polanco
11560 Mexico D F Mexico

International Thomson Publishing GmbH
Konigswinterer Strasse 418
53227 Bonn
Germany

International Thomson Publishing Asia
221 Henderson Road
#05-10 Henderson Building
Singapore 0315

International Thomson Publishing—Japan
Hirakawacho Kyowa Building, 3F
2-2-1 Hirakawacho
Chiyoda-ku, Tokyo 102
Japan

1 2 3 4 5 6 7 8 9 10 XXX 01 00 99 98 97 96 95

Library of Congress Cataloging-in-Publication Data

Shames, Karilee Halo
   Creative imagery in nursing / Karilee Halo Shames.
     p. cm. — (Nurse as healer series)
   Includes bibliographical references and index.
   ISBN 0-8273-6394-X
    1. Imagery (Psychology) — Therapeutic use. 2. Visualization —
Therapeutic use. 3. Holistic nursing. I. Title. II. Series.
   [DNLM: 1. Mental Healing — nurses' instruction. 2. Imagination.
3. Holistic Health — nurses' instruction. 4. Psychiatric Nursing.
WB 880 S528c 1996]
RZ401.S49 1996
610.73'01'9 — dc20
DNLM/DLC
for Library of Congress

94–39827
CIP

INTRODUCTION TO NURSE AS HEALER SERIES

LYNN KEEGAN, PhD, RN, Series Editor

*Associate Professor, School of Nursing,
University of Texas Health Science Center at San Antonio
San Antonio, Texas
and Director of BodyMind Systems, Temple, Texas*

To nurse means to care for or to nurture with compassion. Most nurses begin their formal education with this ideal. Many nurses retain this orientation after graduation, and some manage their entire careers under this guiding principle of caring. Many of us, however, tend to forget this ideal in the hectic pace of our professional and personal lives. We may become discouraged and feel a sense of burnout.

Throughout the past decade I have spoken at many conferences with thousands of nurses. Their experience of frustration and failure is quite common. These nurses feel themselves spread as pawns across a health care system too large to control or understand. In part, this may be because they have forgotten their true roles as nurse-healers.

When individuals redirect their personal vision and empower themselves, an entire pattern may begin to change. And so it is now with the nursing profession. Most of us conceptualize nursing as much more than a vocation. We are greater than our individual roles as scientists, specialists, or care deliverers. We currently search for a name to put on our new conception of the empowered nurse. The recently introduced term *nurse-healer* aptly describes the qualities of an increasing number of clinicians, educators, administrators, and nurse practitioners. Today all nurses are awakening to the realization that they have the potential for healing.

It is my feeling that most nurses, when awakened and guided to develop their own healing potential, will function both as nurses and healers. Thus, the concept of nurse as healer is born. When nurses realize they have the ability to evoke others' healing, as well as care for them, a shift of consciousness begins to occur. As individual awareness and changes in skill building occur, a collective understanding of this new concept emerges. This knowledge, along with a shift in attitudes and new kinds of behavior, allows empowered nurses to renew themselves in an expanded role. The Nurse As Healer Series is born out of the belief that nurses are ready to embrace guidance that inspires them in their journeys of empowerment. Each book in the series may stand alone or be used in complementary fashion with other books. I hope and believe that information herein will strengthen you both personally and professionally, and provide you with the help and confidence to embark upon the path of nurse-healer.

Titles in the Nurse As Healer Series:

Healing Touch: A Resource for Health Care Professionals

Healing Life's Crises: A Guide for Nurses

The Nurse's Meditative Journal

Healing Nutrition

Healing the Dying

Awareness in Healing

Creative Imagery in Nursing

C O N T E N T S

Preface, xv
Acknowledgments, xvi
Introduction, xviii

Part I   INTRODUCTION TO IMAGERY IN HEALING, 1

Chapter 1   *Seeing with the Inner Eye: Use of Therapeutic Imagery in Nursing, 3*

Dynamics Of Chronic Pain, 4
   Pain As A Body Messenger, 5

Guiding the Healing Journey, 6
   Barriers to Self-Awareness, 7
   The Need for Self Re-Evaluation, 8

The Nurse As Health Educator, 9

The Power of the Mind, 10

The Power of Images, 11
   Sources and Effects of Images, 13

Right Use of Intuition, 15

The Healing Power of Emotions, 17

Summary, 20

References, 20

Chapter 2   *Introductory Experience and Insights: Sample Guided Imagery Session, 21*

Analysis of Session, 32
   Post-Session Thoughts, 32

Definitions of Terminology, 32
  Imagery, 32
  Therapeutic Imagery, 33
  Guided Imagery, 33
  Interactive Guided Imagery ᔆᴹ, *34*

General Concepts Relevant to Sample
Imagery Session, 34

Summary, 36

References, 36

Chapter 3 **Hypnosis and Imagery: Historical**
Perspectives, 37

Comparison of Hypnosis and Imagery, 38

Hypnosis, 38
  Use of Hypnosis Across Time and
  Culture, 39
  The Ancient Greeks, 39
  The Middle Ages, 41
  The Renaissance, 41
  Cartesian Dualism, 42
  The Eighteenth and Nineteenth
  Centuries, 42
  The Twentieth Century, 43

Carl Jung: Major Contributions to Symbolic
Value, 43
  The Symbolic Value of Dreams, 44
  Instincts and Archetypes, 45
  Exploration of Consciousness, 45
  The Role of the Psyche, 46
  Symbology and Mythology, 46
  Cultural Images, 47
  Images, Emotions, and Reason, 48
  Fear of the Unknown, 48
  Initiation Rituals and Symbology, 49

The Impact of Jungian Thought, 49

The Work of Clarissa Pinkola Estes, 50
  Symbology in Storytelling, 52
  Stories As Food for the Soul, 52

Modern Times: Creative Visualization and
Guided Imagery, 53

Summary, 55

References, 55

Part 2   *CLINICAL USE OF IMAGERY IN NURSING PRACTICE, 57*

Chapter 4   *General Usage of Imagery Techniques: Basic Clinical Applications, 59*

Role of the Nurse Using Imagery: "Beyond Ordinary Nursing," 59
   Empowerment, 61
   Nurse As Healer, 62
   Clinical Uses of Imagery, 63

Imagery Terminology, 64
   Relaxation, 64
   Mind-Body Connection, 65
   Psychoneuroimmunology, 65

Evolution of Imagery Terminology: A Timeline, 66
   Ancient Times, 66
   Scientific Revolution, 66
   1900s, 66
   PNI Research, 67
   National Institutes of Health: Candace Pert, PhD, 68
   Further Definitions, 69
   Image, 70
   Imagery: Connections Between Senses and Images, 70
   Visualization, 71
   Therapeutic Imagery, 71
   Guided Imagery, 71
   Hypnosis, 72
   Interactive Guided Imagery^{SM}, 72
   The Guide, 72
   Inner Advisor, 72

Where To Begin: Imagery Procedure, 73
   Tension/Progressive Relaxation, 74
   Countdown, 74
   Eye Muscle Tightening and Relaxing, 75
   Pleasant Memory Technique, 75

Deepening: After Initial Relaxation Response, 76
   Breathing, 76
   Inner Sensations, 77
   Inner Body Tour, 77

Finding One's Special Place, 77
  Clinical Applications for a Special Place, 79
  Practical Applications, 79

Quick Uses in the Clinical Setting, 81
  IVs, 81
  Pain Medications, 81
  Antibiotics, 81
  Anticoagulants, 82
  Oxygen, 82
  Healing Image, 82
  Ideal Images, 82

Dealing with Fear and Anxiety, 83
  Tapes for Patients, 83
  Working with the Breath, 83
  Counting with the Breath, 84
  Working with Fear, 84

Summary, 84

References, 84

Chapter 5   Intermediate Clinical Applications:
**   Individualizing Imagery Experiences, 87**

Review: Meeting the Inner Guide, 87
  Introducing the Inner Guide, 88
  General Guidelines for Inner Guide Work, 88
  Considerations When Accessing Inner Guide, 91
  Guiding Clients Through Emotional
  Experiences, 92
  Suggestions for Practitioners, 93
  Advancing Your Skills As Practitioner, 93

Intermediate Imagery in the Clinical Setting, 93
  Advice for Beginning Nurses Using Imagery, 94
  How To Make Time For Imagery, 95
  Developing Open-Mindedness, 96
  Legal Considerations, 97

Other Uses of Imagery, 99

Birth-Related Imagery, 99
  Antepartum, 99
  Labor Imagery, 100
  Postpartum Imagery, 100

Affirmations and Imagery, 101

Habits, Addictions, and Imagery, 102
  Imagery and the Addiction Process, 105

Imagery in Oncology, 106
　Simonton Technique, 106
　Imagery Rehearsal, 108

Suggested Imagery Techniques for Pain, 108
　Breathing, 108
　Working with the Image of the Pain, 109
　Glove Anesthesia Technique, 110

Where to Start, 111
　Intensity Scale, 111

Dialogue with Symptoms, 112
　Pattern Recognition, 114
　Metaphors of Pain, 114

In The Face of Loss, 115

Final Thoughts: Creating Sacred Space, 118

Summary, 119

References, 119

Chapter 6　**Creative Imagery: Advanced Clinical Applications, 121**

Working with Life Transitions, 122

Parts Work, 122
　Regression with Inner Guide, 124
　Healing Another Part: The Inner Child Work, 125

Danger: Planting Images Can Be Hazardous to Health, 126

Re-evaluation of Past Trauma (Reframing), 127

Age Progressions (Rehearsal), 128

Spiritual Nursing Care, 129
　General Spiritual Growth, 129
　The Healing Circle, 130
　Past Life Regressions, 130
　Higher Sense Perception, 131
　Contacting Physical and Nonphysical Guidance, 132
　Creating Healing Teams, 133
　Avoiding Negative Influence, 135
　Imagery in the Face of Death, 136
　Autoimmune Imagery, 137
　Beyond Fear, 138
　Anger and Health, 138
　Playing Detective, 139
　Spiritual Uses of Imagery, 139

Healing of the Etheric Body, 140

Oneness with the Universe, 141

Summary, 141

References, 142

Part 3   INTEGRATION INTO NURSING PRACTICE, 143

Chapter 7   Interviews: Nurses with Imagination, 145

Introductory Ideas of Nurse/Imagery Specialists, 146
    Special Considerations, 148
    Exercise, 149
    Body-Mind Nursing, 149
    Utilizing Client Resources, 150

Summary, 170

References, 170

Chapter 8   Nurse, Heal Thyself: Beginning the Journey, 171

Where To Begin: Initial Steps for Nurses, 171
    Codependence Issues, 171
    Reprogramming: Enhancing Life Quality, 174

Creative Imaginings, 175
    Changing-the-Mind Channel, 175
    Visual Affirmation, 176
    Decisional Affirmation, 178

Whole-Person Nursing Care, 179
    Setting Boundaries, 179
    *Setting Boundaries with Clear
    Communications, 183*

Helpful Hints, 185

Summary, 186

References, 186

**Chapter 9   Weaving the Healing Web: Initial Steps,
Reassurance, and Helpful Hints, 187**

Nurses: Weaving the Healing Web, 187
    *Nurse-Weaving: Introducing Imagery to
    Colleagues, 188*
    *Nurse-Weaving: Enticing Patients with
    Imagery, 189*
    *Weaving Teamwork in the Health Care
    Environment, 190*
    Sacred Weavings, 191

The Web Grows, 192
Doctors and Nurses, 193
Allied Health Professionals, 193
The Family, 193

Helpful Hints, 196
Special Precautions, 196
Creative Nursing, 198
*Honoring Religious/Philosophical
Orientations, 199*

Summary, 200

Reference, 200

Chapter 10   Imagery: Seeing the Nurse As Healer, 201

Nursing As Sacred Work, 201

The Wounded Healer Archetype, 202

Nursing's Special Challenge, 203

Secretary's Commission on Nursing Report, 203

Curing, Caring, and Healing, 204

Healing Rituals, 204
The Hero's Journey: Initial Phase, 205
The Hero's Journey: Transition Phase, 205
The Hero's Journey: Return Phase, 206

The Nurse's Journey, 207
Become Your Own Hero, 207
Bandura's Studies, 207
Nursing Modeling Theory, 208

Summary, 213

References, 214

Appendix: Resource Guide, 215

Index, 221

PREFACE

This book is intended to introduce nurses to the increased healing potential available through incorporating therapeutic imagery into nursing practice. It explores imagery from a historical and holistic perspective, provides examples of actual imagery sessions, and explains how nurses can begin to use this tool for a variety of medical conditions.

In the early chapters, sessions are used to illustrate key concepts. In chapter 1, the topic of imagery is explored as the nurse introduces the idea to a hypothetical client. Chapter 2 is largely devoted to an uninterrupted session with Suzanne (the hypothetical client), followed by key concepts for that chapter. In chapter 3, the historical basis for imagery is presented.

Chapters 4, 5, and 6 describe beginning, intermediate, and advanced techniques of imagery, complete with vignettes and case studies. Chapter 7 tells stories of different nurses who have incorporated imagery into their healing practices. In chapter 8, the nurse who is new to imagery is presented with methods to begin her self-healing journey and become adept in imagery work. Chapter 9 provides special hints, and chapter 10 envisions nurses as healers using the imagery process. An Appendix of additional resources concludes the text.

Author's Note: To simplify and equalize gender decisions in text, the author refers to the nurse-healer as "she" and the client/patient as "he" whenever feasible and appropriate.

A C K N O W L E D G M E N T S

The author wishes to gratefully acknowledge the contributions of other health professionals who have popularized therapeutic imagery for health enhancement, notably the triumvirate of nurse-imagery healing specialists from northern California who so beautifully model collaboration in their teaching endeavors: Susan Ezra, RN; Jan Maxwell, RN, BA; and Terry Miller, RN, MS. Much of the material presented here has come through these delightful women, particularly in chapters 4, 5, and 6. These women have all taken the art of imagery and woven it into the tapestry of nursing in their own joyful ways.

In addition, the author also gratefully acknowledges Terry Miller and Susan Ezra for providing rich editorial expertise. Special thanks to the nurses interviewed in chapter 7.

Likewise, special gratitude is offered to another empowering example of nurse collaboration, Lynn Keegan, RN, PhD, and Barbara Dossey, RN, MS, for their inspiring work and contributions to therapeutic imagery through BodyMind Systems and their many published contributions.

Much appreciation also goes to the medical and philosophical experts who have contributed to the fields of hypnosis and imagery recently, notably: Richard Shames, MD (for writing *Healing with Mind Power*, and for supporting nursing's transformation in so many ways); Joan Borysenko, PhD; Larry Dossey, MD; Jeanne Acterberg; O. Carl Simonton, MD; Lawrence LeShan, PhD; and Kenneth Pelletier, PhD.

The author deeply appreciates the work of the cocreators/ directors of the Academy for Guided Imagery, Martin Rossman, MD, and David Bresler, PhD, who have enriched the practices of countless health professionals through sharing their knowledge about imagery.

Finally, the author gratefully acknowledges Delmar Publishers for its visionary insight in creating the Nurse As Healer series (especially Deb Flis and Bill Burgower) and Lynn Keegan, PhD, RN, for sharing her warm and enriching editorial expertise and for her gracious support as series editor.

This book is further dedicated to the 2.5 million nurses of America. May it tickle your fancies and ignite your imagination for the new age in nursing that we usher in together.

I N T R O D U C T I O N

Can you imagine a world filled with peaceful communities and partnership, a place where people have learned to truly hear each other's point of view, and where mutual respect is a way of life? If so, you already possess a tool powerful enough to help this vision become reality. You are using your imagination.

Though not everyone can readily conceive of a peaceful, loving planet, most of us can easily worry about the future. Have you ever pictured yourself having your worst fears coming true? Your most desired fantasy? These imaginings are far more common.

Having the ability to worry demonstrates the capacity to envision something that has not yet happened. This ability to fantasize future outcomes is a powerful gift, and is perhaps unique to the human species. Were we to consciously channel this process into constructive change, the world could indeed become much healthier.

We have witnessed the benefits of technological medicine, as well as its detrimental side effects. Though modern science has helped to conquer many illnesses, millions of people are still plagued by chronic debilitating diseases for which conventional medical treatment has little to offer.

As nurses, we attempt to inspire people to heal. As long-standing patient advocates, nurses have joined other healing professions to actively explore the advantages of nontoxic, natural therapies, particularly those that stimulate the life force, build a strong immunity, and inspire a more positive outlook.

One such practice, steadily gaining in popularity, involves the use of creative visualization and guided imagery. Creative visualization and guided imagery use the power of the mind to potentiate healing of the body.

Nurses can teach clients to access their inner guidance using the personal symbolic language of their own mental pictures. They can further support this process by providing a safe atmosphere for relaxation and receiving inner guidance, and through assisting clients to value their images and feelings.

One major use of imagery is to help people fully connect with their inner resources. We know from experience that in times of crisis it helps to look inward, perhaps to reflect upon one's situation, or to seek guidance from the creative source, whatever we believe that to be. As health practitioners, we can encourage our patients' growth by teaching them the importance of utilizing their inner-generated pictures.

Images are potent because they move us easily, allow ready access to that which might be hidden from consciousness, and help us to integrate the information we receive for beneficial purposes. For example, when we see a great painting, witness a breathtaking dance, or view a magnificent sculpture we are moved to feel in a way that defies description. Images evoked for healing purposes can elicit an equally powerful, if not greater, response.

As nurses, we strive to offer our patients the most comprehensive care, tending to the body, mind, and spirit whenever possible. We understand that each of these dimensions can play a major role in the prevention of disease.

Creative visualization and guided imagery are very practical tools for nurses to use because they are noninvasive, inexpensive, and fun. Working in this manner, nurses can use their creativity, intuition, and imagination, thus enhancing their nursing experiences while supporting the patient's journey toward wellness.

Creative visualization and guided imagery are modern versions of ancient medicines. A return to these ancient techniques helps restore a sense of balance and connection to humanity. A new era is dawning in health care. The medicine of the future will hopefully be less invasive and more humane, with practitioners helping clients to mobilize their personal resources for self-healing.

Nurses are already in a prime position to promote health education in our role as patient advocate. Understanding and utilizing mental imagery is one additional way to prepare for the transformation.

Increasingly, we health providers are likewise recognizing the inherent benefits of taking good care of ourselves, so we can feel better, increase our stamina, and provide healthy models of empowerment. Through the use of relaxation and imagery techniques, we nurses can access our deepest dreams. We are then more adept at facing challenges in our personal and professional lives.

This book, *Creative Imagery in Nursing,* is designed to inspire nurses and other health care providers to understand the inherent value of these tools, to learn to teach them, and to use them wisely with clients. It is also intended to support the transformation of nursing into new roles as powerful and knowledgeable practitioners. Lastly, this book may further awaken nursing's limitless imagination, so that we can create more joy in all aspects of our lives and inspire greater health for all humankind.

INTRODUCTION TO IMAGERY IN HEALING

1

SEEING WITH THE INNER EYE: USE OF THERAPEUTIC IMAGERY IN NURSING

The focusing power of attention never fails. It is the secret of success. Concentrate . . . Then go after what you want.

Parmahansa Yogananda, 1946

As nurses, we often have the opportunity to work with people as they deal with pain and discomfort. Through the use of imagery, we can utilize our creative inner resources to assist with our client's healing process. The following is an example of one nurse's imagery work with a client in pain.

Suzanne

She sat in the examining room bent over in pain. I had agreed to meet with her for this initial visit to see if we could arrive at some understanding of what it was that hurt so desperately inside of her.

Suzanne had already been evaluated by a general practitioner, as well as some local specialists. She had even sought help at one of the most renowned medical treatment centers in the country. There just seemed to be no relief in sight for this thin, wispy-framed woman.

"Suzanne," I uttered calmly, "you have attempted thus far to get to some answers about your chronic pain in very traditional ways. You've been on pain killers for quite a while, to the point where many of your other systems are beginning to reject this approach. Correct me if I'm wrong, but I think you feel satisfied that there is nothing wrong with any of your major systems." She nodded in agreement.

"It's possible that you have some rare disease or syndrome, but all attempts to find something pathological have failed. If there is indeed a serious problem, it is highly elusive and extremely persistent. Would you agree with this assessment thus far?"

She looked up from the chair with a sad, pouting face and nodded. At 38, she seemed worn out and tired. She looked older than her years, as people in chronic pain often do. I knew she must feel very discouraged, and silently feared for her mental stability at this point.

DYNAMICS OF CHRONIC PAIN

In my twenty years of practice, I have worked with many clients in this state. They have tried what seems to be everything conventional medicine has to offer, with little success. Often, they crumble under the weight of their nameless burden, and either take out their frustration on themselves or those close to them. Either of these choices invariably leads to further demoralization and loss of self-esteem.

As nurses, many of us have come to understand the intensity value of pain. When people reach a state such as Suzanne typifies, one of two things usually occurs. Either they muster all their inner strength to accept their lives, making decisions that enhance their coping abilities, or they perish—physically, mentally, emotionally, spiritually. In other words, they make decisions on the cellular level either to survive or to further degenerate and eventually die.

Much of nursing's endeavor centers around exploring the former decision, aiming to enhance the life force whenever possible. We must often direct the client to address the pain on a physical level initially through proper medical evaluation. Likewise, it is almost always our goal to help others find reasons to live and to be productive.

Pain As A Body Messenger

Consider the analogy that every person is a treasure chest filled with special gifts, if they could just find the key. The key is within their possession, though they may not understand this and often we must sift together, as nurse and client, through the debris of their broken lives to find that key. To do this, the client must be encouraged to view pain from an entirely new perspective.

Our bodies come equipped with feedback mechanisms that support our health. When we become out of balance, perhaps excessive in some way, sooner or later the body will begin to register the effects of that imbalanced living. For example, we nurses have often monitored our patient's acid-base balance, with the understanding that sometimes a slight change in pH can signify impending death. This is also the case with other imbalances. If one ingests alcoholic beverages to excess, there is a progressive deterioration in one's capacity to function. If one ingests food to excess, there can arise the inability to digest. Each of these conditions is met with messages from the body, warning signals that a state of dis-ease is progressing.

When we heed the warnings, the body goes back into a more comfortable state, a state of ease. However, when we ignore the messages, the body speaks progressively louder in its attempts to call our attention back to the source of discomfort.

Pain is one such body messenger. It can be so subtle initially that only the most sensitive, aware person would notice it. That person can respond quickly, taking time to reflect upon the meaning of the discomfort. "Oh, I almost forgot. It's time to take my medication." "I'm beginning to feel a little dizzy. Perhaps I'd better sit down for a few minutes." Most people, however, do not heed the subtle early warnings.

In modern life, this delicate warning system has dramatic competition. With sirens screaming in the streets and horns blowing in our ears, it is increasingly difficult to pay attention to all the warnings. We have adapted by stretching our capacity to endure these noises, to the extent that in many ways we are less than responsive to even the screaming sounds. As for quiet whisperings, they carry little impact for hectic lives.

There is a great danger in not responding. The word *responsibility* is actually related to one's "ability to respond." When we become numb to the calls around and within us, it takes progressively louder warning to get our attention.

It is the same with bodily pain. It can start off as a soft, inner calling, but because most of us are well-trained in denying our feelings, we pay little attention to those subtle warnings. Soon, the pain becomes more insistent. We feel insulted. After all, we have much that is important to do and never quite enough time to do it all, so we must prioritize.

Another limiting factor, affecting our willingness to listen, is the expectations we have developed in our fast-paced culture. Because we are accustomed to instant gratification and fulfillment, we are less patient with enduring a process that can be comparatively time-consuming. Often to really hear and understand the body's messages, we must give ourselves time to listen without all the distractions that are so prevalent around us. Cultivating that kind of attunement is a lesson in patience for most of us. Yet regarding the concept of pain, it is a lesson well worth the learning.

GUIDING THE HEALING JOURNEY

For all of these reasons, a healing journey can feel frightening to our patients. For some, it might even be likened to a descent into their personal hell. It must, therefore, be supported by loving, kindly guidance.

Those engaged in this powerful healing work must have done their own "homework." To be willing to support another's journey as a guide, one must first have undertaken this journey oneself. We may not have arrived at our final destination, but to be believable, we must have faced our fears to some degree.

When we examine the word *healing*, we discover that it is derived from the Greek word *halos*, which means hale and hearty; it is also related to the words *whole*, *healthy*, and even *holy*.

A holistic framework allows us to work with a whole-person belief system, one that supports body-mind-spirit integration. To help people heal or become whole, we must help them become aware of all of the parts of themselves, including those they have neglected, rejected, or denied.

Barriers to Self-Awareness

Why do people neglect, reject, or deny parts of themselves? To answer this, we must remember that we have developed sophisticated defense mechanisms to help us survive life's traumas. Our psychology background as nurses taught us about the many and diverse coping skills we utilize daily just to exist and fit into our culture. In addition, we tend to resort to personally chosen coping maneuvers to adapt to our unique conditions.

Some of our adaptations can be considered healthy, in that they promote a sense of being whole, of feeling empowered, and of loving ourselves. At times, this ability to be flexible can save our lives. However, many of our chosen adaptations can be life-affirming initially, then progress into unhealthy, life-denying habits, especially if we do not let go of them after the need to resort to them has passed. It is these parts of ourselves that require ongoing review to remain in a state of balance and wholeness, rather than disease.

To illustrate this, consider the child who was often beaten into submission by an alcoholic parent. Years later, this person might well have learned not to talk back or to say anything about how he's feeling. However, long into adulthood, we may find this same person in the professional arena, attempting to work with an aggressive (sometimes alcoholic) supervisor. The adaptation syndrome is still in effect, even though the situation is quite different.

No longer a helpless child, this person could speak out, calling upon coworkers and superiors, even contacting social services if necessary, to maintain his rights. However, having learned to be subservient and submissive long ago, he may be prolonging the abuse, not only for himself but for coworkers, by refusing to be assertive. In this demeaning process, one is progressively devalued, allowing fears and past pictures to rule, destroying potential confidence and contributions.

The Need for Self Re-Evaluation

Most of us seem to have areas in our lives that are in need of re-evaluation. If we are afraid when someone raises his voice, terrified to ask for what we need, or abusive to others unnecessarily, it is usually a result of childhood programming that needs to be replaced with a more empowering attitude for a mature adult.

We can become empowered when we do the tedious yet invaluable work of dragging the skeletons out of the closet and exposing them to the light, where we can see how little weight they carry. We must admit that they exist if we are to heal.

Denying parts of ourselves can lead ultimately to a sense of dissatisfaction, or disease. *Disease* can literally mean to be ill at ease, and when we are chronically ill at ease in our bodies and our lives, we are much more apt to become sick.

Long-term *dis-ease* can undoubtedly account for much of the chronic illness in our population. Therefore, as nurses we must consider the effects of negative coping behaviors on health. We can sit by our patients' bedsides, or see them in our offices, and offer them keys to help themselves unlock those fearful, forgotten places.

"Suzanne," I began, "I would like for us to approach your situation in a slightly different manner for the time being. Are you willing to try some simple, noninvasive maneuvers to see if we can get to the bottom of your condition?"

She looked at me askance, as if she were seeking more details without having the energy to speak. I continued, "What I mean is, I would like to start as if we were at the beginning of a very exciting adventure, and that you and I were copilots on a mysterious journey.

We have agreed to work together for a common cause, in this case to uncover some secrets that have thus far eluded the team on this venture. Can we agree to fearlessly approach this mission, knowing that there is little to lose but a great deal to be gained if we succeed? Success will be measured solely through our own interpretations of our endeavors, and certainly by how we feel about ourselves and our contributions at the conclusion. What do you have to say about this?"

I waited quietly for her response. "I think I understand what you're suggesting," she commented. "You think that I could change my pain by changing my attitude. Is that it?"

"Yes, Suzanne. I believe it's worth launching a new effort at this point, using all the knowledge we have gained thus far to help us go further. I think you may have gotten bogged down in fear and disappointment, and that together we might be able to alter the direction of our investigation."

"So, how do we start?" she asked curiously.

"Suzanne, I would like to take you through a relaxation experience in which I offer some relaxing suggestions while you are more comfortable and less stressed. In that state, we can access some material from your subconscious, if you will. We can bypass the exhausting effort of trying to figure everything out with the mind and allow for some inner visions to surface. Does that make sense so far?"

She nodded as a slight smile began to curl up the corners of her previously pouting mouth. "I know what you're doing. You want to hypnotize me into telling the truth."

THE NURSE AS HEALTH EDUCATOR

At this point, needless to say, I had to spend some time talking with my client, making distinctions between medical hypnosis and some of the more gentle forms of guided imagery and visualization. Basically, in the creative visualization process, the client provides much of the direction. The nurse guides the client, using her creative skills to make this adventure meaningful for the client.

To be powerful in this role, the nurse can use all the knowledge she has gathered about people in general and the client in particular. It is a very creative endeavor. I see it as a cocreation, a mystical joining of nursing and spirituality. When we return to simple, time-honored practices, nursing revives a long-lost, and much-needed, art form.

Even when the nurse provides a guided meditation experience, she is very attuned to the mental, emotional, and spiritual needs of the client. Each time this tool is used, it can be used in a totally different and equally powerful way. It can be surprisingly fulfilling for the client and also for the guide. Nurses will definitely enjoy their work more as they reclaim hands-on, open-hearted traditions in their practices. They will also be more prepared in the expanded role of health resource guide.

THE POWER OF THE MIND

Many popular books in demand today speak directly to the issue of the power of the mind (see Appendix). Most of these books agree that the mind can be our most powerful ally, as well as our most powerful enemy. One prominent theorist, Kenneth Pelletier, even titled his book *Mind As Healer, Mind As Slayer* (1979).

Great theorists and motivators such as Napoleon Hill (1989), Og Mandino (1983), and even the more current medical theorists Bernie Siegel (1986) and Gerald Jampolsky (1979) agree that channeling mind power is the secret to success. Whether your goal is financial gain or a greater sense of well-being, positive thinking is the most direct route to achieving your goals.

Many studies have amply demonstrated the placebo effect. The power of the mind can easily overshadow the benefits of chemical medicines and even psychotherapeutic counseling. In fact, Deepok Chopra, an Indian physician trained in the United States, has questioned the negative mindset so prevalent in modern doctors (1989). He coined the term *nacebo effect* in reference to the phenomenon whereby a patient is told by his doctor that he has two months to live, so the patient complies and dies in two months.

Dr. Chopra could not help but wonder whether the doctors were right a great deal of the time, or whether their negative predictions had planted seeds that found fertile ground in the overwhelming fear of their patients. Rather than defy their doctors, the patients seemed to surrender to the belief of the doctor, thereby fulfilling the negative prophesy.

America's most studied and well-known psychic of the early twentieth century, Edgar Cayce, wrote many books related to natural healing modalities. His ideas were so influential that an organization was dedicated to researching them—the Association for Research and Enlightenment, or A.R.E., with headquarters in Virginia Beach, Virginia. A medical clinic is located in Phoenix, Arizona. It was Mr. Cayce's belief, as documented in numerous readings from the A.R.E. library, that the mind is the builder and the body the result.

These examples could continue indefinitely, so extensive is the literature relating to the mind-body connection. Entire organizations have sprung up worldwide to make this information and research accessible to many.

What is important is to understand that the mind is our greatest tool and that we can each become students of mind power, learning to harness the power of the mind to heal the body, and, ultimately, our lives.

THE POWER OF IMAGES

According to *Webster's New World Dictionary* (1967), an *image* is a mental picture, a representation of something that can be real or imaginary. When children wake up with frightening nightmares, it does little good in the moment to tell them the fear is unfounded, that the creatures they envision do not exist.

To the mind, an image is powerful whether or not it has a physical counterpart. The images we invoke in our minds can be terrifying or life-sustaining. Fortunately, we have the ability to control our thoughts and to focus on life-affirming images.

Consider the example of a pilot shot down over enemy territory in World War II. In captivity for over a year, he watched as his fellow captives disintegrated in body, mind, and spirit. The deplorable conditions sickened the majority, yet he persisted in thriving.

Man's Search for Meaning (Frankl, 1959), a classic book written about this topic, explores the attitudes that allowed people to face life after the atrocities of war had devastated all that was meaningful to them.

Dr. Frankl found that there is a place within us that senses our connection to the greater good, the creative source of our lives, whatever we choose to name that source. Those who survived war, and thrived, managed to tap into that eternal essence, that place of peace inside themselves.

This survival depends upon an ability to create positive images in the mind and to hold the firm belief that these images will become a reality. The loved ones waiting at home, the potential for a new and even better life, the fulfillment of dreams; these are the images that keep people alive.

Today, there is a burgeoning field known as psychoneuroimmunology. It is a result of many years of study in the interrelationship between the mind and the body's immune system. There is vast evidence that holding positive images boosts one's immune system and that thinking negative thoughts, with their concomitant unsettling images, weakens our defenses.

Carl Simonton, MD, and Stephanie Matthews-Simonton (1978) are pioneers in this field, having worked with cancer patients for many years using positive images to mobilize their defenses against the disease of cancer. They encouraged their patients to look inside, to pay attention to the positive images they saw, and to change negative images to improve their ability to cope.

In our culture, the advertising industry has capitalized on the obvious impact of images on the human psyche. For example, there has been enormous emphasis on images of physical bodies. We see countless beautiful bodies on magazine pages, coupled with products being advertised. Why? We see these images because the industry knows how our minds respond to images. Our minds correlate these images and make purchasing decisions based on the advertising trick. "Smoke cigarettes and you too will be a handsome man with a beautiful woman on each arm." These are Hollywood-inspired images, projected from an advertising executive's mind onto the screens of millions of people's minds across the world.

How true are these images for you? Images are most meaningful and helpful when they arise from a person. The creative mind has the capacity to conjure up very detailed images. For this reason, many of us find that television and movies will never replace the magic of reading.

This is not to underestimate the impact of media images on the average person, for that impact is immeasurably powerful. However, when we read about characters in a book, even with the most comprehensive description, our minds create the characters as we read. This internally generated creation can touch us very deeply. It is a different experience from working with images painted from someone else's imagination; those images are more like second-hand pictures.

Children are often natural imagers. We can see them playing in the yard, talking to imaginary friends and later telling us very tall tales about things they "saw." However, most of our children have been educated in highly linear thinking. Our children are encouraged earlier and earlier to forget about imaginary friends and to learn to memorize facts. They (and we) have often been told that we do not really see what we see or are not really feeling what we say we feel. After many such episodes, the child has learned well to disregard his own feelings and imaginary world.

The child instead learns that his outside voices carry more weight than his internal ones. He begins to relinquish his power to heal, as well as his ability to imagine. Consequently, this may be the beginning of illness.

Sources and Effects of Images

Images can come to us through many senses. We tend to think that to use imagery, we must see things perfectly in our mind's eye. In truth, an image is a thought with some sensation attached. We may see a picture, but it may not be as clear as it would be in real life. We may also, however, get a feeling, or smell or hear something. These are all images, as shaped through the various senses.

When I tell you about lemon juice, you may have a physiological response. You may or may not see a picture of lemons or juice, but you may feel an autonomic response to whatever your image is.

If I were to ask you to imagine picking a nice yellow lemon from a tree, cutting it open, and squeezing the juicy pieces one at a time, like most people you would probably begin to respond physiologically. If I further encouraged you to imagine taking that lemon juice and pouring some onto your tongue, and tasting the sour taste, you would likely pucker up and salivate. You have not really tasted lemon, but your body is responding in a sensory manner to the image.

Similarly, when I remember my grandmother's kitchen when she baked, I am flooded with many sensations. I can see her standing there, four feet ten inches tall, with her flowered apron and her rolling pin in her hand. I can see my grandfather sitting at the table, making sarcastic comments about her chicken soup.

I can hear a faint blaring of the television always on in the next room, and I can feel the cold Pennsylvania wind blowing through the cracks in the old kitchen door. I can hear her sing-song voice vibrating in my ears, always finding something upbeat to talk about.

I can easily taste those chocolate chip cookies as they melt in my mouth, and I can feel a tug on my heart for the wonderful values she gave me and the loss in my life since her death.

One image can carry a depth of meaning and can evoke many powerful emotions and sensations all at once. The thought of a nuclear bomb going off can arouse major physiological responses in my body almost immediately. My throat feels dry and scratchy, my voice feels shaky, there is a sensation of gloom and dread around my heart, and I feel the rage of a mother lion protecting her cubs from impending danger.

Sometimes the images can be symbolic. Cave drawings from prehistoric times tell of the lives that were led and attempt to convey feelings about those lives. They may not accurately reflect the outer world, but instead reflect the inner process.

We definitely experience physiological responses to our symbols. The autonomic nervous system is responsible for unconscious responses. In humans, the imagination is involved in this process more than other animals. We have the mechanism to filter distortions of sensation, to alter them with our emotions and our thoughts. Our response to art is filtered through our emotions. In fact, the language of the arts is to create and convey emotions. We also have physiological reactions to thoughts and images. When we think about someone we have loved and lost, we may trigger a grief response through the image we hold mentally.

This gift, the ability to feel raw emotion without thinking, is a result of our right-brain (intuitive) activity. The right-brain response is unfiltered by thought; it is quick, insightful, and intuitive. It may also be symbolic, less structured by reality, and more imaginative.

"Suzanne, I don't want to hypnotize you. Remember, I have invited you to join me in creating something positive. The images I would choose may not necessarily be meaningful to you. I have had different life experience, education, and therefore different beliefs than you might have. I'd like for you to come up with your own images. Imagery is powerful because there is more emotion accessed through symbols than words, but the symbols must be personally meaningful to you."

I watched as Suzanne's face reflected puzzlement. The nurse must always be aware of subtle changes, no matter how insignificant they may appear to be. That level of attunement, that use of intuition, has always been one of nursing's greatest strengths.

RIGHT USE OF INTUITION

According to Napoleon Hill, author of the best-selling book *Think & Grow Rich* (1960), intuition is an enhanced state of perception in which all the other senses are so finely attuned that a synergy is created. In synergy, the sum total is greater than the contributions of each of the parts. Intuition, therefore, is a high-level attunement through alignment of our senses.

The shaman of ancient cultures was a most sensitive healer. He paid attention to all the clues, striving to be in touch with divine guidance to support the healee's recovery. Though a part of everyday life, the shaman was distinguished by his ability to "walk between two worlds," that of the physical and that of the spirit. This delicate dance required total concentration and dedication of the shaman's innate wisdom or intuition.

In modern life, today's "shaman" walks between two worlds as well. Modern life dictates that we be very attentive to day-to-day details. Yet, the shaman is devoted to maintaining that connection with the higher self, that which supports our journey toward our fullest realization as human beings. The shaman knows when to speak and when to remain silent, when to share visions and when to listen to the person's dreams.

This delicate balance requires a firm footing. As nurses, who guide people on their healing journeys, we must have our feet firmly planted on the ground, yet always be listening to that inner voice, that which knows all things and reveals all things. It is in this act that nursing's spiritual nature is most remembered. The intuition of both healer and healee is important to the process. Intuiting is definitely a spiritual practice.

In every culture, from the most ancient to modern day, there has been a name for the inner knowingness we possess. Some call it inner wisdom, the three-million-year-old healer, intuition, or God. Whatever our beliefs, we have all crossed rocky channels and been guided through some connection to the divine.

When we browse through nursing history, we can see that our roots as nurses are firmly planted in religious thought. Many of the early nurses were monks or nuns. As we explore the holistic model, we can see how nursing's empowerment today depends upon our willingness to remember those aspects that distinguish nursing from other groups. Our spiritual core and our attention to emotion are such areas.

As I watched Suzanne's face cloud over in puzzlement, I knew that she was wondering about the importance of emotions in healing. I had just stated that imagery's power lay in its strong emotional impact.

"Suzanne, you look confused. Did something I say disturb you?"

"Well, it didn't disturb me, but it did make me wonder. Why is it so important to my health that I feel strong emotions? I don't see the connection. It seems that I've spent most of my life trying not to be so overwhelmed by feelings. I've always been told that I'm too sensitive for my own good."

THE HEALING POWER OF EMOTIONS

As a nurse and therapist, I am always relieved when a client wants to know more about the mind-body connection. Certainly, I consider one of my major roles to be that of health educator. As a counselor, I have come to understand the importance of the role of emotions in healing.

Holistic practice is the perfect place to address this conceptual framework. It is with a great pride that more and more nurses are turning to this fulfilling concept. As holistic nurses, we can help clients claim *all* parts of themselves, to learn to accept and honor them all. Emotionality is one such valuable part.

Emotion is a subjective response to a person or situation. It can relate to various concepts in our everyday life, including feelings, passion, sentiment, humor, mood, attitude, beliefs, opinions, and views, to name a few. Some holistic practitioners consider the emotions to be one of the major components of holism (i.e., body-mind-spirit-emotion).

Combining these different components is the key. In my private counseling practice, I have the opportunity to sit with people for an hour that is devoted exclusively and wholly to that person and his process. Invariably, the medical condition can be found to have some connection in the emotions.

When I serve as a willing collaborator, the person is allowed to feel supported in looking at emotional material that has been long buried, or repressed. This material sometimes takes on very graphic representation in the form of bodily ailments.

For instance, I worked with a client who was experiencing bilateral tendonitis of the elbows. Initially I was slightly apprehensive about helping someone with these limitations, because

I had not done this before. I wondered what I, as a psychological counselor, could offer.

I asked the client to show me where the pain and discomfort was, and then to explain to me everything that had led up to that situation. He told me that it had occurred initially several months ago, when a cord of wood was delivered and dumped in his driveway. He had to move the entire load of wood three times to get it stacked in the desired location.

I knew he lived alone, and carried some resentments towards his ex-wife, so I asked him what his thoughts were while he was stacking that wood over and over. His recollection, not surprisingly, was that he was angry and hurt at having to do all the work.

In reflecting upon his symptoms, I spontaneously had a vision of his pummeling someone. I found myself asking him who he wanted to hit, to which he responded with a nervous laugh. He then told me that he was furious at his ex-wife and another man who had been slandering him.

When he realized that he was very angry with these two people, it became more apparent to him why both of his arms wouldn't heal. He was carrying tremendous energy toward them both. It was my recommendation later, by the way, that this particular client pull out his "poison pen" (he loved to write nasty letters) to release these toxic feelings. He did, and was better able to relax and heal.

It certainly does seem that the body speaks to our lives, and reflects our lives sometimes very poignantly. Consider the phrases "I was scared stiff"; "I don't think I can stomach this"; or "He's the most hardheaded person I've ever met!" Would it surprise you that the first person had arthritis at some point, the middle had ulcers, and the third had constant headaches?

Conversely, our emotions can be a wonderful ally when we are journeying toward health. Dr. Gerald Jampolsky (1979) initiated an organization called The Center for Attitudinal Healing in Tiburon, California. This center is dedicated to helping people strengthen their emotional bases for their healing endeavors. For two decades, families challenged by life-threatening illnesses have been learning to express feelings and to experience more positive emotions, even in the midst of crisis.

After all, whether or not people are cured, or even live, isn't always the issue. What is often most important is to upgrade the quality of life. It seems that in our culture, a great fear and denial surrounding death exists.

In many other cultures, there is a greater understanding and acceptance of the life/death cycle. As nursing returns to its roots, we must allow people to grieve and mourn more fully, perhaps even create more rituals surrounding birth and death, and to inspire our patients to be more accepting of all parts of life. This is wholeness too.

"Suzanne, your emotions are one of the very beautiful parts of you, and what makes you so special. I honestly believe that our emotions are our inner selves calling to our outer selves for some awareness. I don't think we can go too far astray if we learn to listen to the messages behind the feelings. Not feeling emotions can be dangerous.

"We have all tried it the other way. We have denied our feelings to the point where it seems as if it is in vogue not to feel. I'm concerned about the unwillingness to feel our emotions.

"I believe that denying our feelings allows them to grow into something unmanageable. They become poison that overtakes us, polluting everything not only inside us, but also around us. In this sense, perhaps it is our feelings that most guide us towards a healthier existence."

Suzanne seemed relaxed and more at ease after all this dialogue. She then informed me that her younger sister was a nurse, and was not enjoying her nursing work because of the heavy application of medications and technology.

Now I realized that Suzanne sought not only pain relief for herself, but also was searching for new hope for her sister's plight. She asked several questions related to visualization history and technique, which I assured her I would answer after we tried some gentle relaxation and guided imagery. She relaxed as we began the imagery experience.

SUMMARY

As nurses, we are often in a position to support our clients on their journeys toward a sense of wholeness and increased understanding. This dialogue reminds us of our creative potential as both health educators and healers.

References

Chopra, D. (1989). *Quantum healing.* New York: Bantam Books.

Frankl, V. (1959). *Man's search for meaning.* Boston: Beacon Press.

Hill, N. (1989). *Think and grow rich.* New York: Ballantine Books/Napoleon Hill Foundation.

Jampolsky, G. (1979). *Love is letting go of fear.* Millbrae, CA: Celestial Arts.

Mandino, O. (1983). *The greatest secret in the world.* New York: Bantam Books.

Pelletier, K. (1979). *Mind as healer, mind as slayer.* New York: Delacorte Press-Seymour Lawrence.

Siegel, B. (1986). *Love, medicine, and miracles.* New York: Harper & Row.

Simonton, O.C., & Matthews-Simonton, S. (1978). *Getting well again.* Los Angeles: J.P. Tarcher.

Webster's new world dictionary: Compact school and office edition. (1967). Washington, D.C.: World Publishing Company.

Yogananda, P. (1946). *Autobiography of a yogi.* Los Angeles: Self Realization Fellowship.

2

INTRODUCTORY EXPERIENCE AND INSIGHTS: SAMPLE GUIDED IMAGERY SESSION

Imagery is not only a set of tools for healing, but for preventing illness and living the highest quality daily life. It can help you create a life of meaning, of purpose, and of wellness.

Martin Rossman, 1987

After introducing the concept, the nurse can proceed with the imagery experience by staying very involved with the client's process. In the following pages, the nurse guides the client through her initial experience using imagery.

Suzanne was sitting comfortably in a big, soft chair with her feet flat on the ground and her hands relaxed on her lap. I encouraged her to take several deep breaths, breathing fully in with the nose and blowing out with the mouth. For several minutes, we focused on relaxation through deep breathing, with me breathing fully and deeply in conjunction with her. I encouraged her to ignore any sounds or to incorporate them into her state of relaxation.

"When you breathe in, see yourself pulling in strength and wisdom with every breath. You can also envision that you have openings in the center of the soles of your feet, and as you breathe in, you are drawing in fresh, powerful energy from the earth. You are feeling very connected to the earth and its healing energies. You might even envision roots going down each leg, through the opening in your feet, and burrowing down, down into the earth.

"You may also see another root coming from your tailbone, from the tip of your spine, and growing down into the center of the earth. All three of these roots meet at the earth's core, where they hook into the center of the earth. In this way, you feel very grounded, very supported, very connected to the earth.

"As you breathe in, Suzanne, you pull energy from the center of the earth up, up, up into your body. You feel a sensation of warmth, you may see light filling every vein, every artery, every organ. As you exhale fully, let go of any stress, any pain, any discomfort. Breathe in strength, and wisdom, and joy . . . blow out any pain, any sorrow, any negativity. Breathe in courage, blow out fear. Breathe in love, blow out tension. Use your breathing to recharge yourself, to let go of anything that no longer serves your highest good, and fill those places with love, and joy, and strength."

In glancing at Suzanne, even with the lights dimmed, I could notice a sense of peace surrounding her, an easing of the fear and tension that she had been carrying for so long and that had been compounded by her shallow breathing and sense of despair. Her face now appeared less anxious.

"Suzanne, I would now like to invite you to go to a special place, a place that has special meaning for you. It might be a place you have been to before, a place that holds special meaning and memories for you, a place that feels safe, and secure, and nurturing. It might also be a place that is created from your imagination, a place you would love to go to.

"Imagine that you have found this wonderful spot to rest in, away from all the distractions and chaos of your normal life. Take a few slow, deep breaths and bring your awareness to this place of peace. As you breathe in, be aware of the sights that surround you, and notice in great detail the scene before you. See the colors, the shapes, the objects with a crystal clear vision. If there are any life forms, notice what they are and breathe in their special beauty.

"As you breathe in even more deeply, notice the smells. Breathe in the fragrances, notice if there's any wind, and feel the sensations from the environment surrounding you. See yourself in this beautiful and peaceful place, and allow your senses to be filled with the wonder and enchantment of a child.

"If you enjoy sitting by the ocean or a babbling brook, imagine that you are near one. If you feel more comfortable in the mountains or the desert, imagine that scene surrounding you. Feel free to embellish your special place until it is filled with wondrous sights in every direction. If there are certain sacred objects you would like to have there with you, objects that make you feel more comfortable, see them with your inner eye.

"Feel your body relax even further, as if you were shedding off weeks of stress and tension. Feel the layers peeling off you as if the tension were a coat you had been wearing and were now relieved to dispose of after a long, tedious journey.

"Suzanne, from this very relaxed place, I'd like to ask you to scan your body. Start with your toes and wiggle them, move them, tighten the muscles, then let them relax. Now move up to your ankles and move them around, tighten them, then have them relax. Keep breathing and allow your body to gradually descend into a deeper state of relaxation.

"Tighten your calf muscles, then relax them. Tense your knees, and thighs, and the muscles around them, then let them relax. Now move up to your pelvic area. Tighten the muscles in the entire area— your gluteus muscles, your abdominal muscles, all the supportive muscles for your pelvic cavity. Now let those go, and feel a deep sense of relaxation and release. Now move on to the muscles in your waist area and chest; tense the muscles of your chest and upper back. Feel them get tight and hard, then let go and feel them relax. Remember to continue to breathe deeply. Every breath in fills you with strength, courage, and wisdom; every breath out releases any fear, any pain, any discomfort.

"Now move up to the muscles of your neck. Let your head hang, allow the muscles to be loose, limp, and relaxed. Slowly, ever so slowly, move your head around in a circle, breathing and feeling the muscles as they let go. Feel the warmth and energy moving through this area as the muscles relax and the blood flows more fully. Feel your shoulders relax, allow them to roll softly and gently. As the shoulders move in a circle, feel the muscles of your back and neck relax even further. Feel all the muscles as they release. Thank those muscles for supporting you in all that you do.

"Feel your head as it rolls around on top of your neck. Your head feels comfortable and free as it floats around effortlessly. Wrinkle your brow, clench your jaw, then release, feeling the muscles as they relax. Your face feels smooth and at peace. Your head feels relaxed and at ease. Your entire body feels relaxed and loose.

"Now scan your body from head to toe. Notice if there are any areas still in need of release. Pay attention to any places that might need to relax a little more, any areas where there is still a sense of holding. Breathe into those areas, and as you breathe in and out, feel the muscles relax and let go. Breathe out any fear, any pain, any tension. As you breathe in, draw in strength, courage, and wisdom. Blow out any pain, any hurt, any fear. Breathe in love.

"Now, Suzanne, in this very relaxed state, take several more deep breaths. Each breath draws you more fully into a state of relaxation, a place of peace, a time of power. Feel your body relaxed and rejuvenated, be aware of your feet on the floor.

"All that exists at this moment is your breathing, the sense of connectedness you feel with the earth's healing energy, with all beings and life forms, and with your highest self. As you breathe in and out, you feel more and more in touch with your inner guidance. Pay attention to any visions you might see, any messages you might hear, or any information given to you in this relaxed and peaceful state.

"In fact, this is a good time to ask your inner guidance, or higher self—whatever you call the creative life force—for some information to support your efforts on this healing journey."

At this point, Suzanne seemed deeply relaxed and at peace. She looked almost like someone who was asleep, except that she was sitting erect in a chair and seemed alert and responsive to suggestion.

"Now picture yourself resting, perhaps in your pleasant spot, in perfect weather, surrounded by bliss. You are comfortably curled in your special place when you notice a figure slowly moving towards you. It is a creature, either human or otherwise, that seems very much a friend to you. It may come in the form of a wise older person, a guru or religious figure, or an animal. Perhaps it is someone you know or someone you have known. It may be a person or figure that carries special meaning for you.

"Slowly, gracefully, gently, the form approaches and sits across from you. You are still in a very relaxed and restful state, and the being looks into your eyes. As you meet its gentle gaze, you feel enveloped in a pink cloud, and you are overcome with a feeling of being protected and loved. You feel very safe, very special, and very cared for.

"You become aware of a deep sense inside you that this being has come to serve you in your search for healing. As you look into its eyes, you see a love and gentleness that transcends any feeling you've had prior to this time. There is a deep calm inner knowing that this person or creature was called forth by your innermost wisdom to bring you a message. You are certain that the message is crucial to your well-being, and that paying attention to this information could actually save your life.

"With a deep reverence, you sit up straight and peer into the eyes across from you. For this moment, nothing else exists, or matters. You know you have come all the way to this special place to receive the gift this creature promises.

"Now, Suzanne, take some time to commune with this creature. Look deep into its eyes and ask the questions that your soul has yearned to have answered. Allow them to flow effortlessly forth from your heart. Let your mind be still, and from that place of inner peace, allow the questions to bubble up from your hungry soul.

"Keep the mind at rest. Let the thoughts arise as tiny bubbles from the inner recesses of your being, and watch them float to the surface of your awareness. Allow your heart to speak its concerns to this wise reflection sitting opposite you, knowing that you have come to this special place of peace for a healing to occur. You are feeling fully prepared to hear whatever is given to you, knowing that the gifts offered are coming from a deep wisdom that serves your highest good.

"Sit in communion now for several minutes with this kindly guide and breathe in its wisdom and love. Allow yourself to feel bathed and nurtured in its caring protection, and trust that you will be given everything you need to restore your sense of wholeness and wellness. From this sacred moment, call upon all the powers available to support you in your growth. Ask to be given whatever it is that will help you to understand what you've been going through, and why it has been given to you. Ask for the lesson in the experience of pain and discomfort, and sit peacefully as your understanding becomes filled with insight . . . "

Suzanne took several slow deep breaths, and I breathed deeply alongside her to support her process. At this point, I became silent, content to breathe deeply alongside her and to allow my peaceful state to enhance her sense of safety and support. I allowed my own mind to be relaxed and invited any images that could serve her on her journey.

After several minutes, I noticed that Suzanne had a warm, radiant smile across her face, and I saw that she was receiving some help with her long-standing health challenge. As I breathed in and out deeply,

I felt very in tune with her process. After some time, I felt inspired to join with her again.

"Suzanne, raise the index finger on your left hand if you need more time to visit." (Her finger went up slowly; I waited for several more minutes before approaching her again.)

"Now, Suzanne, again use the index finger to let me know if you need more time." (Her finger did not go up after a while, and I was comfortable speaking more.)

"This is a good time to say farewell to your guide. Take another minute or two to ask any other questions that remain, then allow yourself to see your guide moving farther into the distance. Before it leaves, you might want to offer it something as a gift, and your guide might also leave you with something to remember it by. See the two of you exchanging gifts and saying goodbye in whatever manner feels appropriate. When you can no longer see your guide, take several deep breaths."

When I saw her take several deep breaths, I began to invite her to leave her special place and to join me once again in the office.

"Now, Suzanne, it's time to take leave from your special place of peace. Take a last look around for today and breathe in the peaceful atmosphere that has surrounded you for this past hour. Draw in strength, and courage, and vision from this visit, and promise yourself that you will come back here whenever you need to replenish yourself. Remember that this personal retreat place lives inside you and can never be taken away. Keep in mind that you can take yourself back to this beautiful and peaceful place whenever you want to return. Trust that it always has been and always will be available for you.

"With these loving, nurturing thoughts, send a fond farewell out and gradually let your consciousness return to the room where you started. Become more aware of your feet being firmly planted on the ground in this room. Feel your feet on the floor, feel the chair under you, and slowly begin to stretch and move around in space. Take some slow breaths and with each breath return more to the room.

After stretching gradually, allow your eyes to open and become aware of some of the objects in the room around us."

Suzanne's Experience

Suzanne stretched, breathed in and out deeply several times, and sat up erect. Slowly, her eyes opened, and she searched for objects to focus upon. In another minute or two, she looked at me with a sense of calm amazement. Her eyes opened wide and she became very excited.

"Wow, that was amazing. I feel like I've been gone for hours."

I sat quietly, waiting for her to gradually come back to this level of reality. In some ways, doing a visualization or meditation is very much like taking a trip; it requires a gradual reentry.

She looked into my eyes, and suddenly seemed to come to life. She was bubbling with enthusiasm, and I encouraged her to first write a few of her most crucial realizations. I handed her a paper and pen, and put soft lighting on for her to write by. After several minutes, she seemed at peace, even more so for knowing that her images were captured for future reference. She had organized her thoughts and was now ready to share.

"I was sitting in the woods, in a special place I used to imagine as a child. It was like many places I've visited since, but then it was a place to escape from the trauma of my early life. I used to go there all the time when my parents were arguing with each other and with my older brother. It was always there for me; it was a place to run away to.

"This time, it was even more lush and colorful than I remembered. There were beautiful trees all around and a creek that was perfectly clear. I found a nice grassy cushion to lie on, and while I was resting at the water's edge, a beautiful deer came up and sat across from me. Though I had seen him before in my visions, he never stayed very long. He was older now, less frightened, and when

I looked into his eyes, I saw a wisdom and compassion such as I have never known.

"I've always loved deer, and even as a child I used to dream that one day I would catch one, and it would live with me forever and be my best friend. I've read that the Indians believe the deer to be a symbol of gentleness. This deer was like the eldest deer, and he reminded me to be more gentle than I've ever been, especially with myself.

"That alone was very important for me. It may sound simple, but I have been very angry with myself and with my body for all the pain I've experienced recently. It seems I've gotten into some sort of blame cycle, and the more pain I've had, the more I've been down on myself. It seemed a vicious cycle was dominating my life.

"The deer looked deep into my heart and asked me why I've been so sad. I told him that I had pain all over in my body and that I couldn't understand what was happening to me. I felt abandoned by my body and had become very angry with it. The pain started last year, and at first it seemed to be behind my heart. It started as a dull ache, then got louder and louder until it felt like a knife in my back. I was aware of it all the time by then, whereas when it had started, it was only an occasional stab.

"I told the deer that it seemed to get progressively worse, even though I was stretching and having regular massages. Eventually I went to see a chiropractor, but my family started insisting that I seek 'regular medical treatment,' so I saw our family doctor. He sent me to a series of specialists, and I feel like I've been on a roller coaster ever since.

"I've spent hundreds and hundreds of dollars I can't afford trying to figure out what's wrong, and I don't feel any closer to understanding. In fact, I have felt more and more removed. It has become a vicious cycle of frustration. I have felt angry at the medical personnel with their smug smiles and their narrow viewpoints. They each seem to only know about their own little field, and no one seems to be able to look at the bigger picture.

"The deer seemed to be a wise counselor. I have long believed in the power of animals to help heal, especially the deer. It was just so perfect that that beautiful deer came to me. What he said was profound."

I waited, knowing that it would take time for Suzanne to gather her thoughts and organize her feelings enough to be coherent. It was obvious that she had experienced a meaningful interchange, and I was eager to hear about her insight. I also trusted her timing.

"The deer told me that I have become overly reliant on the opinions and advice of others. I definitely agree with that. I know that I felt more in touch with myself before all this happened. It seems that I lost confidence in my own abilities to listen to my body. When I was younger, I used to talk to my body parts, especially when something hurt, and pretend that the part was answering me. The deer told me that this 'game' had served me well for many years and that I needed to do something like that before turning all my power over to the 'experts.'

"He said that the body has a language of its own and that I needed to learn to pay attention to what it was saying. Then he said that if I would spend more quiet time with myself when I experience pain, I could get in touch with what the body needs. Lately I've been running off to some health expert everytime I experience discomfort, hoping that someone could relieve my pain.

"The pain pills I've been taking have further obscured the bodily communications. Not only have I been unable to feel the discomforts, but most of these pills have side effects that are uncomfortable. Some are constipating, others irritate the stomach and intestines, and the deer even said that a lot of the pain I've had recently is directly attributable to the medications I'm taking for pain relief. Isn't that a stitch!"

Suzanne smiled at her statements in disbelief, shaking her head. It was an amazing revelation to her that much of her pain was induced by the very pills that were intended to relieve pain. She was even able to find some humor in this, and suddenly she gave a loud belly laugh.

"The deer then asked me to go back to the time when I was first experiencing the pains behind my heart. He wanted me to tell him what was going on in my life at that time.

"At first I couldn't remember, but suddenly I began to feel those pains as we talked, and along with the uncomfortable feelings, I remembered that my husband and I were fighting bitterly around that time. As I began to tell the deer about the fights we were having, I realized that some deeply buried memories were surfacing as well. I saw that when I was the age that my daughter is now, my parents got divorced, and it felt like my heart was broken.

"Through this flood of memories, I realized that I was dealing with some very old issues. I was absolutely devastated when my father left, and I have not seen him since. Not only was I upset about having bitter arguments with my husband, but I was also dredging up memories that were long buried. In addition to the stress of our fighting, I was deeply worried that our marriage would end as my parents had ended theirs, and my daughter would be in the painful position I was in at her age.

"I saw how that buried grief had encased a broken heart and that my present circumstances were causing the pain around my heart to intensify. It all began to make sense to me, and once I saw it, it was easy to understand why I've been feeling so toxic. Just knowing why in itself caused an enormous sense of relief. The dread I've been carrying for months lifted, and I immediately felt lighter and more at ease.

"The deer reminded me to be gentle with myself. He told me that the little girl inside me had a broken heart from childhood and that I needed to tend to that little girl to help my daughter. It is now very clear to me that I need to deal with the old childhood pains to relieve my present distress. Otherwise, I'm contaminating my present with my past and my daughter's life with mine. It feels so empowering to know what's going on, and I now feel certain I can begin to unravel the knots and heal myself."

ANALYSIS OF SESSION

It is important to note here that not every session conveys this much information. Every session is different, depending upon the person guiding the experience and the client.

Post-Session Thoughts

It is important for nurses to remember that there are many ways to access our patients' creativity and inner resources. This book attempts to share information about one specific category of non-invasive, nontoxic therapies.

Imagery is a wonderful addition to nursing practice for many reasons. Patients love it; it is often something they can grab on to and take home. It empowers them by providing a new skill that makes them feel more in control in the midst of crisis and stressful situations.

As nurses, we must recognize that anxiety is a major secondary issue in our treatment plan. Imagery provides a helpful way to assist in channeling anxiety appropriately and in transforming it.

DEFINITIONS OF TERMINOLOGY

This guided imagery session provides one example of how the mind can be used to heal the body. A variety of imagery techniques and concepts are explored throughout this book. To begin to understand some of the many ways in which imagery can be utilized, we will consider some definitions of terms. Many of these words will be further defined as we progress in the work.

Imagery

The use of the term *imagery* refers to a broad concept, as opposed to *visualization,* which is limited to the sight. These terms are often used interchangeably, but imagery is more comprehensive.

Imagery refers to a natural thought process with sensory qualities, usually associated with emotion. We all have internal images that relate to the various senses. An example of imagery can be seen in metaphors and similes, as when one says "I feel light as a feather."

Many well-known philosophers have referred to the power to use the imagination. Consider the following quotation:

> All the works of man have their origin in creative fantasy.
> What right have we then to depreciate imagination?
> (Jung, 1933)

Philosophers are not the only group that has tapped into the power of using images. Recent sports endeavors have combined athletics and imagery to enhance performance. Athletes have recognized the potency of aligning body and mind for a synergistic effect.

Imagery is considered a vital component of all healing endeavors. When we consider the roles of placebo, suggestion, and faith healing, we can see that all cultures incorporate some forms of imagery into their curative endeavors.

In today's world, natural and self-care maneuvers such as hypnosis, biofeedback, and relaxation techniques utilize this concept. All of these tools are useful adjuncts to therapies and also help enhance one's self-awareness.

Therapeutic Imagery

Therapeutic imagery involves taking that natural imagery process and using it in a way that directs the mind towards some beneficial results. It is a comprehensive concept that allows us to use the senses and mind to create whatever it is that we desire, as well as to solve problems and conflicts.

Guided Imagery

Guided imagery is similar to therapeutic imagery. The major distinction is that in guided imagery the subject is led with specific words, symbols, and ideas to elicit a positive response.

Interactive Guided Imagery^{SM}

The term Interactive Guided Imagery comes to us from the Academy for Guided Imagery in Mill Valley, California. According to the Academy literature:

> *Interactive Guided Imagery* is much more than simply having a patient listen to a predetermined script. It is a powerful modality for helping a patient/client connect with the deeper wellsprings of what is true for them at cognitive, affective, and somatic levels.
>
> The guide's role in this process is not to provide better images for the client, but to facilitate an enhanced awareness of the unconscious imagery the client/patient already has, and to help the client learn to meaningfully and effectively interact with this process on their own behalf. This is not only capable of bringing about psychological and physiologic change, it also empowers the patient who learns to use the process. . . .
>
> Therapeutically, imagery has the ability to directly modulate the autonomic nervous system, and the power of imagination can be recruited to promote specific physiological changes as an aid to healing. In addition, many studies indicate that certain imagery techniques may stimulate physiologic processes including the immune responses which may potentially accelerate the healing process. . . .
>
> There are few physical, emotional or behavioral symptoms or illnesses that are not affected to some degree by the mind. *Interactive Guided Imagery* is an effective set of tools that can be used to mobilize the latent, innate healing abilities of the client to support rehabilitation, recovery, and health promotion. (Academy for Guided Imagery, 1982)

GENERAL CONCEPTS RELEVANT TO SAMPLE IMAGERY SESSION

The following general thoughts are intended to convey basic introductory information relevant to the previous guided visualization. First, keep in mind that even with the same two people working together, each day is its own blend of feelings and opportunity, allowing for a great range of experiences. At times, the client may feel rested and relaxed; at other times the client may feel a need to be alone to process his own thoughts and feelings.

As in various other aspects of nursing, the nurse using therapeutic imagery needs to be flexible and allow for a flow of events that is comfortable to the client. There may be times when the nurse feels inspired to be more directive, and other times when she clearly needs to pull back, allowing the person much more space for his internal process.

A nurse, during this experience, might receive powerful images related to the client's situation. At times, it is helpful to utilize this information immediately, sometimes it is useful to share it later, and it may be information that is never spoken about. It is very important in doing this work to allow the client to generate the images to the extent that he can, for his own visions can be the most meaningful to him.

There are times when people do not experience any images. This can occur for a variety of reasons. In some instances, the person cannot stop his own mind-chatter enough to receive inner guidance. A person with this problem may require extra assistance.

The nurse can be more active in terms of providing descriptive images for the client to envision. The client might also try biofeedback and other stress reduction techniques for enhanced muscle relaxation and mental focus. Many audiotapes available for rental or purchase support this process of deep relaxation (see Appendix).

There can even be religious reasons for the inability to see, as some religions prohibit the process of emptying the mind. It is always important for the nurse to be aware of these situations and to respect the client's belief systems above all else.

Another important distinction is that some people are not *visualizers* in the sense that they don't really *see* images. Instead, the dominant sense might be kinesthetic, where a person senses something. They may hear words, voices, or sounds. Taste or smell may also be involved. All of these senses contribute to the experience, even if the person can't describe the experience. Some sensations defy description, just as most feelings do.

In addition to these diversities, the nurse might need to talk more with the client, especially if the person seems anxious (notice the respirations) or uncomfortable (pay attention to skin pallor, perspiration, facial expression). As in other nursing situations, we must pay careful attention to the subtle, often invisible clues that guide us in our endeavors. Whatever we can do or say to put a person more at ease supports the process.

As a brief example, once when I performed this relaxation exercise, I noticed that as we progressed the man had an increasingly worried look on his brow. It was wrinkled, and his face progressed into what I thought might be a frown.

Finally I asked him if there was anything he needed to feel more comfortable, and he reluctantly asked me if this work was in any way related to the work of the devil. I quickly assured him that this work was intended to call upon the highest wisdom available and it had nothing to do with the devil.

He relaxed slightly, then asked if we were calling upon the angels to help. I told him that if that was a comforting thought to him, he was welcome to view it that way. Only then did he seem relieved, as he believed in the help of angels.

In learning to work with people's inner processes, we must exert great care. This work can be delicate because it touches upon the sensitivities of people's cultural and religious programming. It is a great honor to be allowed to touch people so deeply, and we must move gently into tender territory.

SUMMARY

As in other nursing endeavors, we must cultivate a sensitivity and reverence for the sacred work we do. The ability to be gentle yet powerful is part of our greatest challenge as both nurses and healers.

References

Jung, C. (1933). *Modern man in search of a soul.* New York: Harcourt, Brace, Jovanovich.

Rossman, M. (1987). *Healing yourself: A step-by-step program for better health through imagery.* New York: Walker & Co.

HYPNOSIS AND IMAGERY: HISTORICAL PERSPECTIVES

*Imagery has always played a key role in medicine
. . . A major cause of both health and sickness, the
image is the world's oldest and greatest healing
resource.*

Jeanne Achterberg, 1985

When a client is in crisis, we as nurses can utilize the experience as an opportunity to teach. In the following pages, the nurse conveys historical information to further acquaint the client with the use of creative imagery.

Suzanne had enjoyed her initial experience and told me that she wanted to tell her younger sister all about this. We had a few more minutes left in our session, and she asked if I could tell her more about how imagery was discovered. I decided that that would be a fun thing to share, both for Suzanne's benefit and to support her sister's understanding as a nurse. Suzanne sat back in her chair, relaxed and eager to hear more about the historical basis for the use of imagery.

Though I knew I could not possibly tell her everything about the history of imagery, I decided to bring her attention to information that had excited me when I was learning about the connection between images and healing. I told her that this was a selective historical journey, highlighting what I felt might be most intriguing to nurses who wanted to empower their healing endeavors. With this understanding, we relaxed into a gentle exploration of the connection between the use of images and healing.

COMPARISON OF HYPNOSIS AND IMAGERY

Imagery and suggestive therapy are among the oldest and most powerful healing tools. One combination of these techniques, currently known as hypnosis, has become a widely accepted and very powerful medical practice. Though imagery and hypnosis are closely interrelated, we can make comparisons that will be further expanded. *Hypnosis* is a relaxing state of mind with highly focused attention. One can be in a hypnotized state without imagery, but it is not necessarily meaningful (except for benefits of relaxation).

While hypnosis is a state, *imagery* is a language—the language of the unconscious. One can pay attention to images while in a hypnotic state, but one does not have to be in a state of hypnosis to use imagery. In fact, hypnosis is not essential for imagery to be meaningful. To gain a further understanding of these concepts, we will now explore them independently.

HYPNOSIS

Hypnosis relates to an induced, sleeplike state involving motivation, relaxation, concentration, and application. In this state, the person is relaxed and the mind is directed inward.

The word *hypnosis*, however, has gradually gained an unpleasant connotation for many individuals because of the invasive maneuvers often associated with medical hypnosis. For the most part, movie and television representations seemed to have flavored people's concept of hypnosis, often showing something being done to someone against his will or causing him to act in ways that are embarrassing or out of control.

This turn of events has led to a resurgence of the use of images for healing under a variety of new and increasingly popular names. Some of the presently more acceptable terms are: creative visualization, guided imagery, mind power healing, and psychoneurolinguistic programming.

Visualization and imagery are now popular partially because they signify only the use of images and eliminate hypnotherapy. Keep in mind, however, that hypnosis generally refers to the combination of imagery and suggestion, while imagery and visualization refer to the use of images defined solely by the client.

Use of Hypnosis Across Time and Culture

Anthropologists believe that all known primitive cultures used some form of hypnotic process or trance state as part of religious and healing practices. Tribal healers of all cultures have applied hypnotic techniques to promote a deeper connection to the powers of nature. There was little doubt in ancient times that the role of the mind in healing was supreme.

Histories of people of the East convey similar practices relating hypnotic states and meditation. Both ancient and Renaissance thought assumed a spirit or soul existed that ruled over biological and psychological activity. It was thought that the soul lived in the heart area, where sensations were converted to symbols complete with emotional aspects. In fact, the Greek scholar Hermes believed that images held in the mind had physical properties.

The Ancient Greeks

The ancient Greeks used hypnosis to consult the oracles and created "sleep temples" where people were induced into trances by temple maidens. Bodily processes were stimulated through suggestion, touch, and promotion of faith. Sanctuary walls were inscribed with commemorations of miraculous cures, and statues were erected in gratitude.

Healing methods consisted of religious rites, ceremonies, and special formulas that brought forth the miraculous powers of supernatural beings. Healing themes centered around the belief that one could expel the unseen causations of disease.

Healing was ceremonial, often with the patient stating his ailments affirmatively. Treatment consisted of prayers and incantations, along with the administration of remedies which might be augmented through commands, spells, coaxes, and threats. All of these acts held symbolic meaning which served to affect the patient's mental status.

Occasionally, the priest would don a disguise and appear to the patient as a god for that body part, using relics and gestures to chase evil spirits away. Remedies were supplied, often given to the patients by the gods in dreams. In fact, remedies were often ingested with simultaneous verbal affirmation of the prospect of magic and healing.

Indirect cures were obtained following directions received through dreams and visions. Tales of magnificent cures in the Grecian temples of Aesculapius spread far and wide, inspiring a sort of religious fervor that excited the imagination to the extent that cures were more likely. The walls of the dream temples were covered with symbols. A sacred ceremony prepared the patient to approach images of the god for a healing ritual, an act which further fired the imagination and sense of mystery and connectedness to that which is holy. Dreams and visions were interpreted by priests who directed further care.

Aristotle thought that emotion was always inspired by symbolic representation. To his way of thinking, these emotions were either voluntary (reasonable) or involuntary (irrational). In other words, they were either thought out or not deliberate. These ideas helped explain the irrational behavior of people afflicted with fever, intoxication, or madness. In these uncontrolled instances, the imagination ruled with no limits.

Even after the times of Aristotle, thinkers defined images as emotions or movements of the soul. It was thus understood that people afflicted with disturbing images were out of balance in their lifestyles and were, therefore, not of good health.

The Stoic school of thought promoted the belief that emotion was a distortion of nature, not a balanced state of being. Health was equated with a harmonious life.

The Middle Ages

During the Middle Ages it was assumed that imagination arose from the brain. It then affected the emotions, which caused physiological arousal. This was viewed as undesirable, and attempts were made to eliminate imagination.

Fourteenth-century thought included the belief in a connection between illness and evil spirits; evil spirits were often treated with imagery and hypnotic techniques. In the fifteenth century, the universe was understood through connections with celestial bodies and magnetic forces.

These ideas led Franz Mesmer to develop his theory of animal magnetism, which became very popular by the late eighteenth century. Mesmer brought forth a new understanding of both systematic suggestion and the importance of the healer/ healee relationship.

During Mesmer's time, hysteria was a common affliction. It was held responsible for symptoms such as hysterical blindness or paralysis. Mesmer held some rather unorthodox views and conducted some unorthodox experiments. Although he was controversial, he was effective in obtaining cures. Mesmer felt that hypnotic states came from magnetism, and he recognized the importance of systematic suggestion, which has expanded into the work we are exploring today.

The Renaissance

Physicians during the Renaissance felt that the expression of emotions was intended to restore physiological balance. Imagination awakened the organs for a proper response. If this concomitant physiological response did not occur, the state of imbalance would proceed to a state of deterioration.

The power of the image was supreme, even above the perception or the sensation. Because most of the fears at this time centered around the concept of impending death, a dread of dying was considered the most dangerous emotion, setting into motion the mechanism whereby one was increasingly inclined toward morbidity.

In 1621, Robert Burton published *The Anatomy of Melancholy*. This work, with its references to imagination as the source of melancholy, was frequently cited. It was even considered that parents' imaginings during pregnancy could drastically affect the forming embryo. All pathology was believed to have its roots in dysfunctional imagination.

Cartesian Dualism

All this changed, however, at the end of the seventeenth century. Medical science was then dramatically altered by what is known as *Cartesian dualism*. In attempting to prove the soul immortal, René Descartes separated the mind from the body. All that had previously been prescribed to the soul (imagination, reason, passion) was now assigned to the province of the mind.

Anatomical scientists, including William Harvey (1963/1991), who had been unsuccessful in their attempts to locate the soul, lent further support to the notion that the soul was not part of the mechanical structure or process that drives the body. Even the Church favored Cartesian thought, though it could not explain the physiological changes due to imagination. The human was divided into various parts; each part was assigned to a different health practitioner.

Through this dissection of the human and his emotions, thoughts, and reactions, the value assigned to the imagination dramatically declined. After Descartes, people who were untreatable were accused of having problems of the imagination.

The Eighteenth and Nineteenth Centuries

By the mid-eighteenth century, most previous holistic thought was eliminated in favor of mechanistic thinking. Treatment was mechanical. Humans became the subject of rational observation. Those who attempted to revert to the obvious connection between imagination and physiology were ostracized. Those who attempted to reconnect the soul were scorned, even exiled.

Organic illness was explained via Virchow's cell theory and Pasteur's germ theory. All conditions with no known organic cause were classified as nervous disorders, malingering. Physical conditions thought to arise from the mind were characterized as *hysteria*, the mere rantings of idle women. Scientists who attempted to explain disorders of the imagination were invariably ridiculed.

In the late 1880s, hypnosis became scientifically respectable first through the efforts of Hippolyte Bernheim (1884/1993), and later through the work of Sigmund Freud. Although Freud was impressed initially with hypnosis in his practice, he later abandoned its use, causing its mild disrepute.

The Twentieth Century

The twentieth century saw rivalry between various schools of thought, particularly as several thinkers attempted to demonstrate that imagery was theoretically based in physiology, thus causing a connection between imagination and pathology. Mentalism, behaviorism, and structuralism eventually gave way to a period of neglect of the role of imagery.

Hypnosis, however, enjoyed expanded acceptance during World Wars I and II when soldiers responded positively to it after emotional traumas. In 1955, the British Medical Society endorsed the practice of hypnosis in medical school education. The American Medical Association soon followed.

Self-hypnosis, or autosuggestion, became increasingly popular during the last century, expanding into a growing acceptance of related practices, including meditation, affirmations, and imagery for healing.

CARL JUNG: MAJOR CONTRIBUTIONS TO SYMBOLIC VALUE

Another driving influence toward the ultimate acceptance of the value of images came from the contributions of Carl Jung, an analyst who believed deeply in the importance of dreams and symbols. Dr. Jung actually had a dream in which he was speaking directly to the public, rather than to other esteemed doctors, an unusual concept for an analyst of his time. Because of this dream and his belief in the value of dream material, he subsequently oversaw a project that ultimately became a major influence on the general understanding of the importance of images (1964).

Prior to this contribution, this level of information was considered the sacred property of psychoanalysts and other esteemed scholars. However, since the publication of Jung's *Man and His Symbols*, the lay public has become increasingly knowledgeable and sophisticated about dreams, symbols, and rituals.

The Symbolic Value of Dreams

In *Man and His Symbols*, Jung explored the value of dreams in which images are not coherent and logical. He explained that ideas can pass from the logical, rational mind into the subliminal, thus being altered. This process can confuse the waking mind, distorting our original understanding of the thought or image. The associations can vary in intensity and meaning.

He explained how primitive peoples are aware of the psychic properties of nature, a concept that we "civilized, thinking" beings find foreign. Those fantasy connections are relegated to the unconscious storehouse inside, where we forget them in our thought process, but encounter them in our feelings and reactions.

In this dissociation from the mystical realm, modern humans have divided themselves much as the theorists divided our holistic understanding into its component parts. As a result, the combined synergistic effect was lost. No longer do we consider ourselves part of nature's magic, but rather predictable, rational beings. We have forced that which is irrational into some obscure corner.

Jung felt strongly that many dreams present associations that correspond identically with primitive myths and rites. He suggested that these associations are remnants from the human mind of yesteryear and link the world of consciousness with the instinctual.

Jung believed that our minds, like our bodies, possess a long evolutionary history. Human bodies are similar anatomically to other mammals and the psyche can likewise be understood by exploring the various frameworks from other times and cultures. To deepen this understanding, Jung described his concept of *archetypes* or *primordial* images.

Instincts and Archetypes

Jung believed that those who attacked this concept of archetypes or primordial images lacked the ability to comprehend the psychology of dreams and mythology. Jung felt that the *archetype* is a tendency to form representations of a theme with similar patterns but varying details.

He further clarified the relationship between instincts (physiological urges perceived by the senses) and archetypes (when instincts become fantasies, showing themselves in symbolic images). It seemed obvious to Jung that each newborn animal does not create its own instincts individually; likewise, each human does not invent his own human qualities. Rather, instinct is common to certain groupings and categories. As with instinct, the collective thought patterns of the human mind are similarly inherited, functioning in like manner in all humans.

Exploration of Consciousness

Jung observed that many people use the intellectual process of thought to adapt to their lives, while others, who are also intelligent, adapt through *feeling*. He further distinguished between rational feeling and intuition; intuition is irrational and involuntary.

In fact, Jung explored the various ways in which we correlate experience and consciousness in-depth. He distinguished between *sensation* (tells us that something actually exists), *feeling* (informs us as to whether it is pleasant or not), *thinking* (lets us know what it is), and *intuition* (gives us information about its source and direction). These ideas help us to gain a better understanding of our own beliefs.

These concepts are helpful to a therapist, counselor, or nurse, because we must be in touch with our own biases if we are to remain neutral enough to support another person's process. This mutual respect is the basis for any therapeutic intervention.

In working with images, it is crucial that the client's inter-pretations reign supreme. It is very common for a guide to have her own ideas and interpretations, and it is very difficult not to project these thoughts in one form or another. For this reason, it is imperative that those who work directly with people's images and symbology first explore their own subterranean conscious-ness. In this manner, the counselor develops a major asset: to be able to remain in a neutral position.

Images can be coupled with many levels of feeling, sensa-tion, thought, and intuition. Accessing these various levels can be a delicate process of peeling back layer after layer of awareness. This very sensitive work must be undertaken with a great respect for the protective mechanisms that have supported the person's functioning thus far.

The Role of the Psyche

Freud thought that the psyche possesses a special job, that of "cen-sor" to raw, uncomfortable sensation. The psyche often distorts images to "soften the blow." Jung assumed that the images stored at the less-than-conscious level are less vivid, more amorphous.

However, as images rise to the awareness of the person, they become more clear, sharp, and in focus. Hence, they retain a greater meaning for the person, with an expanded sensa-tional component. In working with a client, one must therefore be prepared to allow the emotional expression that can accompany a journey into one's own symbolic representations. The creation of a safe environment allowing adequate time will ensure a greater degree of comfort with the increased affect that may arise.

Symbology and Mythology

Jung addressed the dilemma of the modern scientific mind. Though we yearn for some spiritual, or religious, comfort, modern humans have a need to witness scientific proof before allowing belief to follow. He felt that we need to be free to choose any point of view, whether it be scientific or religious. In fact, it is in this freedom that life acquires personal meaning.

Religious symbols have always served to give meaning to human existence. So-called primitive peoples have received great solace from their beliefs in a connection to some great creative power. The myths, in fact, take possession of the person, driving him to accomplishments that could not be achieved by mere rational thought alone. Myths are made of symbolic representations that have been invented through subconscious processes.

The original mythmakers were the storytellers of each culture, sharing their dreams and fantasies. It is presumed that the Greek tales of gods and goddesses are based on the lives of people who lived before the stories were created.

Cultural Images

Jung felt that there are *natural* symbols and *cultural* symbols. Natural symbols are derived from primitive cultures and their associations with nature. They can be traced back to archaic roots, to images of primitive societies. Cultural symbols seem to be used to express *eternal truths* and are often used in many religions. They have been adapted and changed through conscious evolution, and have become collectively accepted images.

Because these culturally accepted images can carry emotional significance, it is important to honor these representational sensations in working with images. That which is buried, or repressed from consciousness, nonetheless affects the behavior and sentiments of the person. A simple example is the cross, a symbol that immediately calls forth an emotional response for most individuals in today's world. Another is a swastika, which also creates significant and immediate emotional impact.

When images and the powerful forces connected to these images are disregarded, the consequences can be unexpected, even devastating. The person lives with a potentially destructive shadow that can overpower the waking consciousness. Jung felt strongly that the diseases of modern social life were greatly influenced by the repression of that which was less rational, yet mighty nonetheless.

He specifically felt that as the world proceeded to break down into its territories, the shared inner understandings of nature that bound humanity as one were more and more lost. People have become increasingly nationalistic and isolated, and the shared images have lost their symbolic implications.

Images, Emotions, and Reason

What was previously accepted and understood as natural is presently relegated to the realms of the mystical, which is much less accepted as compared to rational, explainable phenomena. Modern humans scrutinize their mental thoughts carefully and are confused when they cannot understand the emotionality with their minds.

Archetypes are images and emotions that exist simultaneously. The image is empowered by being charged emotionally. For this reason, archetypes must be explored within the context of the entire life situation. The image serves to help connect the whole person through the emotions. A powerful example occurs when many people see beautiful representations of a goddess or angels. There is a strong response to the image and the emotional meaning given to the archetype.

Jung felt great concern that in our industrialized society, we have attempted to overpower nature, rather than bridge our nature to the greater nature. In our efforts to be omnipotent, we have overlooked the enormous power within ourselves as a part of the larger natural world.

Fear of the Unknown

Whereas humankind used to rely on the gods to help in times of trouble, we have now made *reason* our god, deluding ourselves into believing that we have been victorious in our conquest of nature. Jung felt that surely we must look at ourselves, especially our dreams and symbols, while simultaneously looking at the world around us, if we are to comprehend the enormity of our symbolic connectedness. We must explore that which is known (conscious) as well as that which is unknown (unconscious).

In our exploration of mythology, we come to understand that the people in the myths, who are often godlike, are symbolic representatives of the whole psyche. This larger picture lends strength to each individual component.

The concept of the *shadow* alludes to that which is hidden, undesirable, not acknowledged. It is in conflict with the ego, which is often depicted in mythology when the archetypal hero and the evil powers confront each other. Jung felt that we should acknowledge this counterforce, using it to become our own master by integrating all parts of the self.

Initiation Rituals and Symbology

Most cultures have some forms of initiation, complete with their unique symbologies, that allow individuals to establish both their own identities within a group and their connectedness to the group. Initiations often center around the theme of death and rebirth, a rite of passage from one phase of life to the next. Jung proposed that the fundamental goal in initiation processes is often to tame the wildness of the juvenile nature. It is aimed at producing a more civilized, or spiritual, connectedness, even though the ritual itself can often be violent or brutal.

Also, these initiations often center around the theme of man's wisdom merging with woman's relatedness, thus creating a sacred marriage. It is when this sacred balancing of male and female energies occurs within each person that each person can be whole and integrated.

It is proposed that these rituals of transcendence with their accompanying symbols represent our striving to achieve unity within us, conscious and unconscious, male and female, for the purpose of fulfilling our most powerful destinies.

THE IMPACT OF JUNGIAN THOUGHT

Though many people have criticized Jung for his lack of material systematization, it is important to note that the material defies structure because it is irrational and mutable. In boldly refusing to submit entirely to the rational, measurable, and purely intellectual model, Jung has made room for a vagueness that allows for new possibilities; at the same time he honors the complex and diverse nature of humanity. Although the model leaves us unable to define every aspect of human existence, it allows for mystery and spirituality, and, ultimately, the goal of assimilation into a more conscious and balanced existence.

Individually, Jung's work greatly inspires each person to work on her own *inner terrain*, to make peace with her shadow side, and to become increasingly conscious of the forces we may prefer to repress, fully knowing that the forces affect our lives most strongly.

Collectively, Jung inspires us to explore the vast interconnectedness of humanity: past, present, and future. The vast contributions of this bold analyst can never be measured; they can only be felt as our understanding of imagery grows.

It was at this point that I noticed a growing question on Suzanne's face. "You seem to have been following this all along. Now I sense a vague restlessness. Is there something missing for you here?"

Suzanne seemed pleased at my observation. "Yes, actually, this has all been fascinating. I've often heard about Jung, but I never understood the connection between his work and health care. I can certainly see how this can help me in my own personal health crisis. I am wondering, however, how this information can really help my sister enjoy her nursing more."

I was excited by her interest, so I decided to take it to the next level of Jungian thought. "Suzanne, there is a phenomenal book that just came out in 1992 by Clarissa Pinkola Estes, a Jungian analyst.

"She has done a most remarkable job in translating the value of Jungian thought into meaning for the daily lives of women. Because 97 percent of nurses are women, we are challenged by the same issues that most women face. Let me tell you more about her work, so your sister can incorporate some of these ideas into both her personal and professional life." Suzanne seemed pleased, so I began.

THE WORK OF CLARISSA PINKOLA ESTES

Dr. Estes believes that our culture has devalued and undermined the feminine nature to the extent that women have lost touch with their instinctual drives. A most unique woman, she comes not only from the viewpoint of a Jungian analyst, but also from that of a *cantadora*, a Spanish storyteller.

Dr. Estes has traveled widely, learning the wisdom of nature from many varied peoples. Educated in ethnoclinical psychology, she combines the wisdom of psychology with women's wisdom as passed down from generation to generation through stories. She refers to the instinctual woman within us all as the "wild woman."

Estes further makes the connection between this gradual demise of woman's connectedness to her wild self and that of humans to the wildness of nature. She explains that wild women and some of the wild animals (wolves, coyotes, and bears) share related instinctual archetypes and that we are all similarly credited with dangerous and malevolent natures, largely through fear and misunderstanding.

Dr. Estes explains that her training in analytical and archetypal psychology enabled her to further develop her stories, but that it was her upbringing that brought them to life. Having come from a long line of cantadoras, she spent much of her childhood with Hungarian and Latin women whose stories came from their lives and the lives of women before them. To these women, stories are part of the healing ritual.

"For nurses, Suzanne, it is crucial that we leave no stones unturned in our efforts to empower our work and our lives. I believe we are facing one of nursing's greatest challenges today, that of integrating our scientific knowledge with our innate knowledge. All of these ideas about the value of symbols apply to our lives as women and as healers.

"When we learn about symbology, we are also digging through our subterranean selves, looking for answers to our lives and our pains. Beneath our consciousness lies integral and amazing knowledge, as Jung said, and when we uncover this information, we as a species are further empowered." (Jung, 1964)

Symbology in Storytelling

According to Estes, the tradition of storytelling is older than the art and science of psychology. It is often a mystical process, and it can occur through the teller entering into a trancelike state. In this sense, the stories come from a less-than-conscious place, complete with meaningful symbology.

Stories paint pictures in the minds of those who listen. They speak to our lives in symbolic and literal ways. They bring to the surface images that have been hidden beneath the veils of our thoughts. They help us to find meaning in every experience.

"Even your pain, Suzanne, is a valuable messenger from somewhere inside you. It may be physical, and it is therefore very measurable and real. It is also connected to the psyche, to the beliefs and experiences that have shaped your life. There is meaning in the pain, and you can access that by allowing your less-than-conscious process to bubble to the surface."

Stories As Food for the Soul

Dr. Estes feels that stories set the inner life into motion. For this reason, we have visceral reactions to the words we hear. Our feelings come to life, whether the stories are ours or someone else's. The experiences that life offers us as humans have much in common, and often we can learn more about own lives through hearing stories about others.

We can use stories as food for the soul (Dr. Estes calls them "soul vitamins"). They revitalize our process of recovery, soothe our broken spirits, and offer a sense of connectedness to all that is or ever was. Mostly, they help us get back on track; they help us find our way home to our truths.

"Suzanne, I can think of no single greater contribution to a nurse at this stage of our professional evolution than to help her return to the source of her vitality. Nursing is undergoing such a rapid transformation right now, and nurses are grappling with issues of personal and professional power.

"Power is the ability to influence change, and nurses are in a prime position to accomplish healthy changes in the evolving health care system. But first, each nurse must find her way home in her own heart.

"Once she remembers the dream, the vision, the image that led her into her chosen work, the nurse can inspire others to be true to their inner guidance. It is a domino effect, and I encourage you to accept this challenge.

"Creative visualization and guided imagery are entering mainstream medicine more and more each day. There are nurses teaching other nurses how to use these tools for pain control and health enhancement. They are also teaching health care consumers how to use these tools for their well-being. These last twenty years have witnessed a proliferation of information for consumers and health professionals regarding the use of imagery."

MODERN TIMES: CREATIVE VISUALIZATION AND GUIDED IMAGERY

Many books have sprung forth in recent years to further promote the usage of creative visualization and guided imagery for healing. *Healing with Mind Power* was one of the first books that introduced self-hypnosis to the lay public (Shames & Sterin, 1978). *Creative Visualization*, a mass-market book on the use of visualization for healing and spiritual growth, met with tremendous acceptance and helped to inspire a massive consumer interest in this tool (Gawain, 1983).

Since then, hundreds of books and tapes have followed suit, awakening the public and health professionals to the value of imagery and visualization (see Appendix).

In Mill Valley, California, Martin Rossman, MD (author of *Healing Yourself: A Step-by-Step Program for Better Health Through Imagery*), and his associate David Bresler, PhD (author of *Free Yourself from Pain*), have established the Academy for Guided Imagery, which has been operating since 1982. Over 5,000 psychologists, clinical social workers, physicians, nurses, and addictions counselors have taken intensive training programs for clinicians in Interactive Guided Imagery. The Academy provides professional certification, as well as annual conferences and on-going workshops with continuing educational credits in national locations.

In later chapters, graduate nurses from these programs explain how they use this information to benefit patient care in private practice and institutions.

More and more, we see health professionals using learning tools that are based on ancient practice and modified for modern living. Creative visualization and guided imagery are presently enjoying a resurgence in interest because they are cost-effective, empowering, and preventive. There is also wide diversity in application of these techniques. These techniques appeal to a large number of people due to the constantly creative opportunities to use them in different ways.

"Now, Suzanne, maybe you have a better understanding of the potential power of therapeutic imagery in your life. I have guided you through a brief process to introduce you to how it feels as a client to use images for healing. Through this experience, I believe you will begin to see ways in which you can incorporate imagery into your own healing, as well as have some valuable new ideas about nursing possibilities to share with your sister."

Suzanne now seemed relaxed and comfortable. Not only did she feel less anxious and more empowered, but she had learned some very exciting things about herself and how the body and mind can work together. She left feeling jubilant and eager to talk to her sister about visualization.

SUMMARY

As we explore historical relationships between imagery and hypnosis, psychology and religion, we become aware of the symbolic and its diversity throughout cultures. Imagery allows humans to use the mind for many goals. It is rich with historical perspective and future possibilities.

References

Acterberg, J. (1985). *Imagery in healing: Shamanism and modern medicine.* Boston: New Science Library.

Bernheim, H. (1884). *De la suggestion.* Reprinted edition: Bernheim, H. (1993). *Hypnosis and suggestions in psychotherapy.* Northvale, NJ: Jason Aronson Inc.

Bresler, D. (1979). *Free yourself from pain.* New York: Simon & Shuster.

Burton, R. (1621). *The anatomy of melancholy.* London: Oxford University Press.

Estes, C. P. (1992). *Women who run with the wolves.* New York: Ballantine Books/Random House.

Gawain, S. (1983). *Creative visualization.* Berkeley: Whatever Publications.

Harvey, W. (1991). *Circulation of the blood and other writings.* Boston: C.E. Tuttle. (Original work published 1963)

Jung, C. (1964). *Man and his symbols.* New York: Doubleday & Co.

Rossman, M., & Bresler, D. (1982). *Academy for guided imagery* (brochure). Mill Valley, CA.

Rossman, M. (1987). *Healing yourself: A step-by-step program for better health through imagery.* New York: Walker & Co.

Shames, R., & Sterin, C. (1978). *Healing with mind power.* Emmaus, PA: Rodale Press.

CLINICAL USE OF IMAGERY IN NURSING PRACTICE

4

GENERAL USAGE OF IMAGERY TECHNIQUES: BASIC CLINICAL APPLICATIONS

Everyone has images; they are basic to the human mind and human nature. They evolved in the human species long before language did.

Jeanne Acterberg, Barbara Dossey, Leslie Kolkmeier, 1994

In considering the possibilities for the nurse using imagery techniques to support the client's progress, we might first ask ourselves to recall the role of the nurse.

ROLE OF THE NURSE USING IMAGERY: "BEYOND ORDINARY NURSING"

In a recent imagery workshop ("Beyond Ordinary Nursing") written and presented by three nurse colleagues who work collaboratively (Susan Ezra, RN; Jan Maxwell, RN, BA; and Terry Miller, RN, MS), participants were given an opportunity to consider their original visions of nursing, then invited to ponder the following words of Florence Nightingale (1859):

> It is often thought that medicine is the curative process. It is no such thing; medicine is the surgery of functions, as surgery proper is that of limbs and organs. Neither can do

> anything but remove obstructions; neither can cure; nature
> alone cures.
>
> Surgery removes the bullet out of the limb, which is an
> obstruction to cure, but nature heals the wound . . .
> Medicine, so far as we know, assists nature to remove the
> obstruction, but does nothing more.
>
> And what nursing has to do in either case, is to put
> the patient in the best condition for nature to act upon him.

We then gathered into small groups to consider several other questions. First, what meaning did these words hold for us? As we explored collectively, we agreed upon some of the following roles for us as nurses: acting as patient advocates and spiritual guides; helping patients connect to nature; inspiring the will to heal; and providing patients with a safe place to examine their lives.

In accepting that it is part of our nursing role to provide a safe and caring place, we could begin to see the value of incorporating noninvasive tools such as imagery. In fact, when we use basic imagery exercises, we most often commence by inviting the client to breathe deeply and to relax. After achieving some degree of relaxation response, we then invite him to mentally go to a safe place.

The second question we considered together was how our vision has changed since we each decided to become a nurse. This activity touched upon some deep feelings for the nurses in the groups. In my group, several nurses felt that the environment has changed significantly and is presently scary to those still practicing traditional nursing within medical institutions.

For others, especially those nurses who have found a way to practice in less conventional settings, there were also changes from their original picture of what nursing might be like, yet they felt more of a sense of expansiveness, as if the vision had grown over the years. These nurses were able to feel empowered, even more positive, about the potential for their professional enjoyment.

The first group of nurses seemed to feel stuck, and described their feelings as "enraged, frustrated, powerless, and limited." We will later explore which components of their nursing experiences might account for such dramatic differences in perception.

A third issue we considered was what we feel patients need the most. There was, once again, a sense of collective agreement as the following answers arose: advocacy, empowerment (nursing holds the space for people to realize they are their own healers), to take more responsibility for their care, preventive education, connection, touch, and to have their basic needs met.

The final question we contemplated related to whether we felt we were able to meet our patients' needs, and if not, why not? The nurses who felt they were not able to meet their patients' needs gave the following reason: turf wars (between doctors and nurses; between nurses and other nurses, especially nurses between shifts; and between various health care providers).

Many nurses felt particularly squeezed by time limitations. All agreed that we need to stay in physical contact with our patients.

Though I was initially surprised to be asked about visions of nursing in a class about imagery, this seemed to be an especially interesting exercise for a variety of reasons. It is always enlightening to be in a group where nurses can speak freely about their dreams and frustrations, and it was even more enlightening because I was not expecting to consider my "nursing issues."

The nurses felt very connected and relaxed after openly sharing feelings, so the exercise provided us with an enhanced sense of intimacy. More important, however, was the opportunity to begin to grasp the many ways in which imagery can enhance nursing work.

Empowerment

What we decided was that our job as nurses is to help our clients make decisions that are right for *them*; it is our challenge to empower our patients. It is also valuable to consider the topic of empowerment at this point so we can be certain that we all mean the same thing when using this popular word.

The word *power* relates to the ability to influence change. When nurses say they are feeling powerless, it seems that they do not feel capable of producing the desired changes in their work environments and lives.

To *empower*, therefore, means to give one an opportunity to make changes, to enable. It can also relate to the ability to find the power within one's self. In their enjoyable book on empowerment, *Empowerment: The Art of Creating Your Life As You Want It*, David Gershon and Gail Straub (1989) define empowerment as "the art of creating your life as you want it."

Other theorists have proposed that empowerment occurs when you have the skills, tools, information, and support with which to make healthy changes. In all of these definitions of empowerment, there is a sense of power ultimately arising from within the individual who feels supported. When we look at empowerment from this common point of reference, nursing is very much concerned with supporting the patients and assisting them in finding and utilizing their own power.

With this understanding, then, it is easier to appreciate the tremendous frustration nurses feel when they do not feel empowered, and when they cannot support the empowerment of their patients.

As nurses, we must remind each other that we are constantly defining who we are, and that as we seek healing for ourselves and learn to empower ourselves through our self-care efforts, we can serve as healthy role models for our patients. Our experiences, in fact, teach us how to help our patients.

Nurse As Healer

These considerations about our role as nurses help to remind us that part of our job is to inspire the health of our clients. To do this, nurses must be actively involved in their own healing process. There are several reasons for this. First, to do our demanding work and do it well, nurses must establish a sense of well-being.

Just as it is difficult to believe the doctor who tells us to lose weight when he weighs 300 pounds (standard cartoon image), as nurses we cannot be very effective in inspiring health if we are not feeling well much of the time.

Also, we learn from our own process. If we are interested in teaching principles of health, we can best learn by using our bodies as laboratories. When we have first-hand experience, we can speak from that wisdom.

In considering the experience of healing, we must also define what we mean by *healing*. In Middle English, the word *hal* refers to the ability to make whole. The Greek word *haelen* likewise relates to the same definition—to make whole.

As nurses, therefore, we empower and inspire our patients by supporting them in their efforts to make themselves whole. This means that people feel healed, or more healthy, when they can accept and relate to all of the components that make them whole. These components include the parts of themselves, as well as the parts of their lives that are affected by their environments.

Nurses can support their clients' healing by helping them to get in touch with the various aspects of themselves and their lives, and to integrate these components into a meaningful and harmonious sense of wholeness. Let us now consider the role of therapeutic imagery in this process, in light of recent scientific investigation into the interrelationships between mind and immunity.

Clinical Uses of Imagery

In their introductory material to the work of the Academy for Guided Imagery, Dr. Martin Rossman and Dr. David Bresler (1982) articulate some of the many uses of imagery in medicine and nursing:

1. Physiologic relaxation

2. Stress reduction

3. Pain reduction and symptomatic relief

4. Enhancing patient motivation

5. Understanding symptoms

6. Empowering the patient

7. Engaging the patient in self-care

8. Tolerating difficult medical and nursing procedures

9. Enhancing patient compliance

10. Stimulating healing responses

11. Insight/affect recognition

12. Finding meaning in illness

13. Deepening patient rapport

14. Reducing patient anxiety and demands

15. Encouraging active participation by the patient

16. Defining emotional needs of the patient

They also list other uses more closely related to psychotherapeutic goals or dealing with addictions. Some of the uses included in this category are: stress reduction; systematic hyposensitization; conflict resolution; values clarification; shift of locus of control and relief of powerlessness; positive suggestion; affirmation; enhanced self-esteem; finding purpose, meaning, and connection; increased creativity and problem-solving ability; modulation of mood through relaxation; decreasing chemical dependency; turning insight into action; access to repressed memory; death, dying, loss, and grieving; role playing techniques; accessing positive inner resources; identifying patterns from family of origin; recognizing projections; strengthening connections and sharing of affect. The varied uses of imagery come after the *relaxation response* has been established.

IMAGERY TERMINOLOGY

Relaxation

The term *relaxation response* was coined by Herbert Benson (1975) to refer to a psychophysiological state in which muscles are relaxed; tension is released; blood pressure, pulse, heart rate, and respirations are decreased; the brain is in the alpha state; and the parasympathetic nervous system is activated.

When the sympathetic system is activated, the fight or flight mechanism is in effect. In the relaxation response, to the contrary, the person feels calm and relaxed.

In examining brain patterns, as a review, the normal waking state is beta. Alpha is a deepened state of relaxation, followed by theta and then delta. When we as nurses assist our clients in achieving states of progressive relaxation, we are helping them to access inner resources that may have been obscured by the high catecholamine levels and resulting anxious state. This process is not new; in fact, it is very ancient. We might consider the relaxation response to be an antidote to stress.

There are a number of ways to activate this response, including progressive relaxation, starting with a relaxed area and visualizing the relaxation spreading; autogenics; tensing and relaxing muscles; and breathing. These will be discussed in more detail after all terms are defined.

Mind-Body Connection

In earlier times, one or two thousand years ago, people intuitively utilized body-mind data. Aristotle (384 BC), for example, demonstrated a brilliant synthesis of the connection between mind and body. Following the time of René Descartes (1600s), however, bright thinkers such as Darwin (1882) and Sir William Osler (1919) exhibited much more fragmented thinking. Cartesian dualism dictated that the mind and the body were independent and operated separately. Modern scientific research, however, has disproved this idea. We will discuss the implications of this split and its effect on modern medicine further.

Psychoneuroimmunology

As nursing undergoes rapid transformation, nurses are being called upon to use more natural methods to support healing. Many of our patients have had traumatic medical experiences and seek more gentle methods to feel better. They are calling upon nurses to provide them with maneuvers that will support their health.

Nurses are beginning to tread more readily across the line between traditional medicine (as it has been practiced since the technological revolution) and alternative medicines (some of which have been practiced in ancient cultures and are experiencing a revival in today's world).

Chapter 3 presents a timeline for the progress of the field of imagery. More recent discoveries have added to the burgeoning body of knowledge relating to body-mind medicine. One such recent discovery is in the growing field of psychoneuroimmunology.

Psychoneuroimmunology is a cumbersome word, but when it is broken down into its parts, it is easier to comprehend:

psycho—related to the brain, mind, consciousness (keep in mind that in ancient times the mind was considered to be the soul)

neuro—related to the nervous system (central nervous system)

immuno—related to the immune system

Hence, the word *psychoneuroimmunology* refers to a science, a rapidly growing field, that shows the interconnection between the mind, the nervous system, and the immune system.

EVOLUTION OF IMAGERY TERMINOLOGY: A TIMELINE

Ancient Times

Remember from our discussion of the history of imagery that in ancient times (300–500 BC) there was shamanic healing and healing temples. The Middle Ages (500–1400 AD) was a rather dark period in the realms of healing. During this period there was a great deal of fear, spurring witch hunts and a general destruction of anything related to the gentle healing arts.

Scientific Revolution

During the Scientific Revolution (1500–1700), René Descartes popularized the concept that the mind and body were separate, not connected. This led to the methods of treatment that worked separately with mental issues and physical illness.

1900s

The 1900s saw a renaissance in the interest in the mind-body connection. Hans Selye wrote about the psychophysiological effects of stress (Selye, 1956). Around the same time period, there arose a renewed medical interest in the field of psychosomatic medicine. Herbert Benson (1975) shared his valuable insights in *The Relaxation Response.*

As the field of holistic health began to make its entrance in the early 1970s, there was a great suspicion on the part of traditional medical practitioners. What was missing for the scientifically minded was a way to convey the concept of mind-body connection without resorting to metaphysics or religion. Psychoneuroimmunology (PNI) provided that missing link.

PNI Research

Using sophisticated scientific techniques, researchers have been able to show that the brain can send signals along nerves to mount defenses against infection. Furthermore, the brain then pumps out chemicals to help the body fight disease. What makes these discoveries even more important is the added understanding that emotions and thoughts can open or close these pathways. Thus, PNI research demonstrates that mental states can definitely affect the course of illness.

Here is a simplified view of how this occurs. First, the mind creates thoughts, or images. These thoughts or images are linked to emotions through centers in the brain. Signals are sent via neuropeptides, which are messenger molecules. Hormonal changes occur as a result of the signals, thus causing a physiological response in the body.

For a simple example of this complex process, consider the physiological effect when I again describe an experience with a lemon: First, with your eyes closed, I want you to create a picture of a lemon in your mind. You might see it growing on a lemon tree, and you go over and pick it from the tree. You put the lemon to your nose, and smell it. Now you take it into the house, put it on a cutting board, and slice it, cutting it in half. The juice from the lemon drips over your fingers.

Now, cut the lemon again, this time into quarters. Pick up one slice of the lemon in your right hand, and put it to your lips. Gently allow your mouth to feel the soft part of the lemon. While you're holding the lemon to your lips, squeeze a few drops of the juice onto your tongue.

By now you may have noticed a physiological response. Most people will experience salivation early on in this exercise that will intensify as the description continues. This is an example of how the mind (thinking of a lemon) sends signals that cause the body to react physiologically (salivation).

National Institutes of Health: Candace Pert, PhD

Research performed in the 1980s by Candace Pert, a neuropharmacologist from the National Institutes of Health, showed that there are direct nerve pathways between the brain and the thymus (where T-cells mature). Neuropeptides (chemical messengers) can be released at the end of these pathways, latching onto immune cells and changing their ability to multiply and kill foreign invaders.

Pert's research explains that this happens through a lock-and-key maneuver whereby the neuropeptide (key) fits into a receptor site on a T-cell and causes a specific reaction on the cellular level.

Also, hormones secreted through brain regulation can affect the cell's ability to fight disease. Nerve fibers in immunologic organs hook up with lymphocytes, the white blood cells that lead the body's battles against infections and malignant growth. Lymphocytes have their own chemical messengers, especially interleukin, which send signals back to receptor sites in the brain.

In essence, the brain is talking to the immune cells. Nerves and hormones carrying messages are activated during stress, depression, or sexual excitement, thus enabling emotions to alter susceptibility to disease.

Candace Pert was at the forefront of this research. In 1973, Pert was among the first to show that opiate drugs have the ability to bind to cells in the brain.

Several years later came the finding that the body makes its own opiate-like chemicals (endorphins). Research has shown that endorphins have the same mood-altering effects as opiate drugs.

Pert, in her studies of neuropeptides (protein-like chemicals which include endorphins), found that they exist in high concentrations in the limbic system of the brain, which is the center for emotions and drives. Thus, Pert concluded that neuropeptides are the biochemical units of emotions.

She later studied the large amoeba-like cells that surround infection sites (macrophages) and found that neuropeptides can latch onto macrophages and redirect their movement. She believed that if each neuropeptide had a different effect on macrophage traffic, moods could influence the way macrophages fight disease. There are 50 or more neuropeptides, and many other nonpeptide brain chemicals, all of which can affect immune response in a different way.

There has been, and continues to be, a great interest in the relationship between immunity and emotion in recent years. O. Carl Simonton and Stephanie Matthews-Simonton (1978) worked with cancer patients, many of whom were terminally ill, teaching them to aggressively visualize the destruction of the cancer cells by the immune system. They also encouraged patients to take more responsibility for their lives and health status, a concept that has received medical criticism for being so untraditional.

The intent is to inspire the patient to examine all parts of his life and himself. As nurses working with natural healing modalities, we must caution ourselves to provide positive models of healing and encourage patients to honor all parts of themselves without making them feel guilty for their illnesses. This is subtle work, and requires that providers first practice on themselves. (Chapter 8 provides nurses with opportunities to begin their own self-healing journeys, using imagery to feel more whole.)

Keep in mind that imagery provides a mind-body-spirit interaction. The biochemistry involved and the emotional component that is connected result from complex interactions between various aspects of a person. For this reason, nurses who wish to utilize imagery as an adjunct therapy to medical treatment should consider undertaking a more advanced study of imagery (see Appendix).

Further Definitions

Because we have been discussing various aspects of healing and exploring how therapeutic imagery affects one's sense of wholeness, we will now clarify certain terms that may already have been mentioned. Some of these may have been defined earlier and are mentioned again in an effort to reinforce the distinctions prior to deepening the concepts through the experiential chapters that follow.

Image

An *image* is a picture; it is a mental representation of something that might exist. It could also be something from the mind only (something imagined, not real). Images are the language of the right side of the brain, the side that deals less with structured thought and more with creativity and instinct.

Imagery: Connections Between Senses and Images

Imagery is considered a natural thought process using one or more of the senses, and is usually associated with emotions. In other words, it is the process of having thought with sensory qualities. For example, one might see the face of a favorite friend in the mind's eye or envision a lovely rose garden and be able to feel emotions and smell the roses. Consider also the person who was badly burned as a child, and years later takes a position as a nurse on a burn unit. Upon entering the unit for the first time and smelling the burnt flesh, she is struck by a profound sense of terror and pain, and runs out crying. She seems to have a cellular memory of her experience, which is brought to life through the olfactory stimulus.

Another example connecting senses with images occurred when a person who had been in the Loma Prieta earthquake in California watched the television reports of the 1994 Los Angeles earthquake. Upon watching the news, she experienced smelling what the buildings smelled like (in her previous experience) when the buildings collapsed around her. This is another example of stored cellular memory where the person has a sensual response to visual images only; this is imagery.

Often people worry about whether or not they can use imagery; whether or not they have the capacity to see pictures. These people might ask themselves whether they can *worry* about the future. The reason for this question is that if one has the ability to worry, one experiences images. To worry is to imagine a future scene and to have an emotional response to it, even though it has not happened.

We all have responses to images. Picture seeing the Statue of Liberty, a graduation diploma, or a nurse's cap. Pay attention to your emotional reaction to these thoughts. These are external images. Images are also internal. Metaphors and stories are also images that evoke response.

Visualization

Visualization refers to the distinct ability to see pictures in the mind's eye; it is imagery involving only the visual sense. For that reason, we have chosen to present the larger and more comprehensive concept of imagery in place of the more limited ability to see. Creative visualization, as popularized by O. Carl Simonton and Stephanie Matthews-Simonton (1978), generally involves encouraging the client to see pictures of the cancer cells being gobbled by the mighty immunodefensive cells. Creative visualization has been shown to be a powerful adjunctive therapy.

Some people do not see pictures in their minds, but they have other types of responses. Sensory/kinesthetic visualizers experience a thought through feelings rather than through a mental picture. Auditory images occur when we close our eyes and hear a favorite piece of music. Approximately 20 to 30 percent of people are not visual imagers. Therefore, the term *imagery* is used to incorporate all aspects of imagination.

Therapeutic Imagery

Therapeutic imagery, therefore, refers to the ability to take that natural thought process and to direct the mind in a creative way, potentiating a positive outcome. It is a very broad, comprehensive term which encompasses most of the words already defined.

Guided Imagery

Guided imagery is also under the category of therapeutic imagery. It refers to a more unidirectional process in which the practitioner leads the subject with specific words, suggestions, symbols, or images to elicit a positive response.

Hypnosis

We have already explored the field of hypnosis in the chapter on history. *Hypnosis* refers to the tendency to induce sleep. Hypnosis refers to a situation whereby the practitioner is quite active in directing the client, and the client is suggestable and in a very relaxed state.

Interactive Guided Imagery^{SM}

The Academy for Guided Imagery in Mill Valley, California offers certification programs in imagery for health professionals, and coined the term *Interactive Guided Imagery*. This process has the capacity to take the client to an equally deep level as hypnosis through eliciting and working with a subject's images, with less directness. In Interactive Guided Imagery, the guide facilitates the process for the client and the client describes and shares images rather than having the guide present images to work with. This process is dynamic, spontaneous, and most empowering.

The Guide

Keep in mind that when you are guiding someone in an imagery experience, your role is to hold the mirror for clients to see themselves more clearly. You help them to access their own images when possible, and you can encourage the images to have a voice. In this way, the client is dialoguing with his innermost guidance. This belief brings up a very important concept, that of the inner advisor.

Inner Advisor

The *inner advisor* is considered the source of inner wisdom. For each person, the inner advisor will mean something slightly different. In exploring this concept, we begin to delve into some very personal beliefs and it is crucial that we abandon our personal agendas to truly serve the client's needs. This exploration borders on the edge of spirituality and involves a person's individual sense of connection with something greater than himself.

That inner wisdom can be seen as a Higher Power, God/Goddess (whatever the patient believes God to be), guidance, Great Spirit, or any of a great number of concepts. Some consider it to be the spiritual sensitivity, deeper wisdom, source of intuition, higher self, collective consciousness, unconditional loving self, one's own truth, and even the sixth sense. It is important for the guide to nonjudgmentally accept the client's belief system and to allow that system to create movement in the direction of greater integration or healing.

Most often, the qualities of the inner advisor include the following: unconditional love, nonjudgmental acceptance, nurturing, wisdom, honesty, compassion, humor, forgiveness, ever-present availability, fearlessness, patience, and optimism. In many ways, it seems as if we credit our inner advisors with the best qualities of a loving parent, or deity. Because the guide is attempting to strengthen this vital connection, the work can be considered quite sacred.

For that reason, a nurse serving as an imagery guide must be certain to align her intent with the highest good. This is also the attitude of any healer undertaking the sacred work of healing. Many nurses who embark on this journey and grow in their abilities as healers find a deep sense of fulfillment and joy in recovering lost aspects of the healing art of nursing.

WHERE TO BEGIN: IMAGERY PROCEDURE

When we help a person to relax, we encourage the mind-body to be in a quiet, receptive, inner-focused state. This state of relaxation sets the stage for a flow of images. It is strongly suggested that nurses undertaking this work start by using imagery themselves. Chapter 8 focuses on the value of self-healing work for the nurse and advises nurses on how to begin using these tools in their lives. For now, we will examine the basic techniques that can be utilized with our clients to practice inducing states of relaxation.

There are a variety of methods that can be used to encourage people to enter into a state of relaxation. These flow in a progression from induction, to deepening, and on to higher level work. We start with what are called *induction procedures.* We will mention only a few simple maneuvers that can be incorporated readily into daily practice.

Tension/Progressive Relaxation

The first technique is *tension/progressive relaxation,* in which we might start with the muscle groups of the feet (or head). Some specialists believe that one becomes most relaxed when working from top to bottom. Others feel that in a progressive relaxation exercise, it is easier for the client to focus initially on the feet.

The idea with this maneuver is to help the client focus the mind on the body, much as the Lamaze method for childbirth does. It is hard to think about the many other problems in our lives when we are paying close attention to our bodies. For that reason, this sort of distraction technique works well.

The client is first encouraged to take several deep breaths and relax. He is then advised to feel his feet on the floor. Next, he is told to squeeze the muscles in his feet and perhaps scrunch his toes and tighten his feet until his feet feel small, perhaps round. Then, the client is told to relax those muscles. This technique serves to focus attention on body parts, one by one, and to make the client very aware of what it feels like when that part is tense, and how it feels to relax that same part. There is often a great sense of letting go with this exercise. The guide then encourages the client to focus on the calves and to tense and then relax those muscles. In a very methodical (hypnotic) manner, the guide helps the client to focus on all major muscle groups and to relax them in succession: the abdomen, arms, face, and so on.

The result is a deep sense of relief, for so many of us have developed unconscious holding patterns in the body, patterns that restrict our circulation and relaxation. Once this process is complete, the more experienced guide can proceed to a more advanced maneuver.

Countdown

Another simple technique is the *countdown.* In this common exercise, the therapist can suggest in a variety of ways that the client count from ten to zero, and that when the client reaches zero, he will be completely relaxed and refreshed. This programmed thought helps to promote a relaxation response which can be further elicited by visual cues, particularly visual imagers. For those people, the guide might suggest a scenario much like the following: "Pretend that you are in an elevator going from the tenth floor to the first. (First be sure that the person does not experience claustrophobia!) On the wall you see the numbers of the floors, and each time the number changes you find that you experience a greater sense of relaxation and relief. When you arrive at the first floor, you will feel thoroughly relaxed, refreshed, and rejuvenated."

There are many variations of this technique, and experience will help the guide find the ones that work best for each client. However, it is always best to review ideas with the client if you are not familiar with his preferences. In this manner, the guide can tailor-design a relaxation experience that will be most helpful and healing for the client.

This aspect of imagery also benefits the guide, or nurse, who usually enjoys returning to the belief that nursing care at its best is highly personalized. Many nurses find themselves revitalized by discovering simple methods to relax themselves and their clients during stressful situations. Most nurses also very much enjoy the renewed sense of creativity that accompanies this experimental process.

Eye Muscle Tightening and Relaxing

While the client is sitting comfortably with his eyes open, he is instructed to either raise the eyes high in the head or focus intently on an object. Doing so results in a certain amount of eye muscle tightening and fatigue, which is then relieved by comfortably closing the eyes. The juxtaposition of the tightening followed by the relaxation encourages the onset of a relaxed state.

Pleasant Memory Technique

The client is comfortably seated and is told to close his eyes. He is encouraged to think back to an enjoyable event, a time when he felt successful and joyful. Reliving this pleasant memory in a safe, comfortable setting often induces the relaxation response.

DEEPENING: AFTER INITIAL RELAXATION RESPONSE

Once a relaxation response has been initiated, the role of the nurse is to further that response, to deepen it to a level that is optimal for allowing the patient to accomplish inner work. The role of the guide is to help establish a sense of safety, which enables progressive relaxation.

Breathing

We mentioned Lamaze earlier as an example of a simple distraction technique. In Lamaze birth breathing, the client is so focused on the breath pattern that she does not have the ability to pay attention to anything else, including the amazingly forceful contractions in her belly. This is a common example of how breathing can help one to relax in the midst of stress.

Another common way to work with the breath is to make the client aware of his breathing pattern, whatever that pattern may be. This is done through simple suggestion ("I want you to begin to notice your breath. Pay attention to the inhalations and exhalations, and notice whether your breathing is shallow or deep. Watch the breath as you focus on it, and notice if there are any changes in the quality or quantity"). This sort of exercise serves to internalize the client's attention and makes the client more aware of his inner world and processes.

The guide can also be more direct, asking the client to take several slow, deep breaths. The client can then be encouraged to use some special kind of breathing (for instance, birth breathing in which the breath is pulled in through the nose and blown out through the mouth). This sort of focus also demands great concentration and allows other parts of the body-mind to relax. Many women have found this cleansing breath to be particularly helpful to ease the discomfort of childbirth. It can be practiced more vigorously to counterbalance other painful experiences.

The breath, besides providing a focus for the mind, promotes the exchange of oxygen and carbon dioxide and allows for a physiological rejuvenation along with the mental and physical relaxation. Exhalation, especially long and deep, stimulates the parasympathetic nervous system. Though it appears very simple, much of the Eastern philosophy (meditation, yoga, and so on) is based on these practices.

Inner Sensations

Another very useful deepening technique is to assist the client in sensing some physiological function, such as the heartbeat. The experience of becoming attuned to one's rhythms is deeply satisfying and relaxing.

The guide might say "See if you are quiet enough to hear or feel your heart beating inside your chest. Perhaps you might feel it as a pulse in your thumb or in your foot. Once you feel it, you can sink into enjoying that sensation. It is the rhythm upon which life depends; see if you can be part of that rhythm. If you can't find it directly, you might wish to imagine it. See if you can achieve a general feel for what it would be like to notice your heartbeat or your pulse, and maybe even to count it."

It is handy to make use of what might otherwise be distracting to enhance relaxation. For instance, if the client has audible intestinal rumbling, have them focus on the inner sensation.

Inner Body Tour

Once the client has closed his eyes and is partially relaxed, encourage an inner exploration, a guided tour through the various organs. The tour might start with the lungs or heart. "From this area, flow outward to all the other tissues and organs. Follow the path of the red blood cells and oxygen as they course through the arteries. Visit the kidneys and the spleen; see the chemical factories in the liver. Enter the control room of the brain. Marvel at the harmonious complexity, all parts working silently beneath the surface."

FINDING ONE'S SPECIAL PLACE

Once the guide has helped the client achieve a state of relaxation, often the next step in imagery is to assist in the creation of a safe place. Keep in mind that some people have not experienced a deep sense of safety in their lives, so we must tread respectfully in learning to guide.

To invite the client to a safe place, we might begin with any of the simple relaxation techniques until he appears to have reached a state of peacefulness. The guide can also ask the client to signal in some way (nod head, raise finger) when he feels very relaxed. Again, this allows the client to feel in charge, enhancing the likeliness that he can proceed to find a place that feels safe. Once he has achieved a sense of relaxation, invite him to go to a place that is peaceful.

The guide can suggest that this place can be real, perhaps a vacation spot or beautiful scene in nature from earlier memories, or imaginary. This is the client's own creation, a sanctuary for that person. The guide can encourage the client to find this place in the mind by suggesting that it is private and peaceful, real or imaginary, safe and secure.

This part of the process can be done quickly. The guide might suggest that the person select one spot only for today, even if they have several places in mind. If the client seems to have difficulty finding a place, the guide must take time to help the person access some idea that is personally meaningful. The guide might say, "If you could imagine a relaxing beautiful place, what would it be like?"

For some clients, the task of achieving a sense of relaxation and peace might be a major undertaking. It is important to honor each person by meeting him wherever he is, and not placing our expectations upon him. If, in an initial experience, all that can be accomplished is to encourage a person to relax some muscles and breathe more deeply, that may be enough for that person at that time.

It is not our agenda that needs to be met; we must always consider that the person is exactly where he needs to be at that moment. Again, part of the creative aspect of this work is to assess where the person is and to encourage healthy motion, rather than pushing and inviting resistance. We are the patient's advocate and ally. By allowing him to feel in control, we offer him a sense of empowerment.

Once that place is located, encourage the person to embellish it with sensory recruitment. In other words, help him to enliven the image by suggesting he consider some of the follow-ing: "What do you notice?" "What is the weather like?" "What do you see, hear, smell?" "How do you feel in this place?" "What time of day is it?" "Which season is it there?"

Tapping into all the senses enriches the imagery. All of these ideas help to bring the sensation of the special place alive, and often the person will become quite descriptive. As he becomes more involved in the description, he achieves deeper and deeper states of relaxation.

Clinical Applications for A Special Place

For clients, going to a special place might be used for a variety of reasons, including for pain relief, for distraction during a pro-cedure, or for anxiety relief prior to surgery.

Caregivers can also benefit from taking the time to go to a special place. In these instances, it allows a place for respite and serves in stress management for nurses and other harried professionals and technicians.

Practical Applications

Now let us consider how the nurse introduces imagery in her daily client contact. The setting can be home, hospital, clinic, industrial, school, or even private practice; for the most part the introduction will be similar.

CASE STUDY | Introducing the Concept to Mr. Jones

Mr. Jones is a 65-year-old patient in a nursing home. He has been confined to a wheelchair for the last thirteen years, following a stroke that left his right side paralyzed. His wife helped to care for him until two months ago, when she injured her shoulder. She continues to live in their nearby apartment and walks over to see him every day after lunch. However, she is no longer able to provide the basic assistance that he has become so accustomed to.

The nurses on the unit have noticed that Mr. Jones has become progressively more demanding and belligerent. Whereas he used to clean his dentures and eat his breakfast every day, he now refuses to cooperate in activities of daily living. He has been complaining about a pain in his hip, and pain medications don't seem to help.

Susan B. is the medication nurse on his wing. She enters his room early one morning. "Good morning, Mr. Jones, how are you doing today?" Mr. Jones groans in response. Susan has been wondering how to help Mr. Jones in recent weeks and suddenly remembers that she could try some relaxation exercises.

"Mr. Jones, I brought your pain medication, but I know it hasn't been working too well for you lately. I have some other things I would like to try to help ease your pain. Would you be interested in trying something new?"

At this point, Mr. Jones responds positively. Susan uses the teachable moment to acquaint him with gentle relaxation. This is a simple example of how the nurse might introduce the topic and seize the opportunity to add basic imagery techniques. Now we will consider several other situations in which imagery can be introduced simply to enhance the quality of care.

QUICK USES IN THE CLINICAL SETTING

There are numerous ways for nurses to initiate changes through use of imagery in the clinical setting. Following are several ideas, supplied by Terry Miller, RN, MS, to inspire nurses to get creative about incorporating imagery into nursing procedures with ease and efficiency.

IVs

When a patient is receiving intravenous fluids, he can envision fluid flowing to every part, removing toxins and flushing them out. The patient can see nutrients providing nourishment to every cell.

Pain Medications

Similarly, the patient can enhance the benefits of pain medication by envisioning its soothing effects as it travels through the bloodstream, sedating any irritated areas and bringing a deep sense of relief throughout. (It is suggested that relaxation be used at the first sign of discomfort; focus the patient on the breath. Imagine the body releasing its natural medicine to all the areas that are tense or uncomfortable. If pain begins to interfere with activity or rest, ask for medication before becoming so uncomfortable that it would be difficult to work with relaxation and the following imagery.)

"Imagine the pain medication to be exactly the strength it needs to be. See, feel, or sense the muscles around the painful area softening and relaxing as you breathe into the discomfort. See or feel the pain medication moving to that area and numbing it as if it deposited a layer of frost.

"Imagine a dial registering a number from 1 to 10 that represents your pain now. See the number come down to your tolerance level. Allow an image to form of a special, quiet, restful place and allow yourself to be there as you rest."

Antibiotics

Some patients like to imagine their antibiotic medication in the bloodstream as hunters stalking their prey. They can envision that the medication stays where the most protection is needed, particularly around burns or incisions, ready to pounce. If more medication is needed, there is an endless supply in the imagination.

Anticoagulants

Likewise, clients using anticoagulating agents can envision their blood becoming thinner, flowing to exactly the right places to prevent clotting. They can see the medication as extraordinarily efficient and relish in watching as it does its magic.

Oxygen

As you take a deep breath, send nourishing healing oxygen into every cell of your lungs, expanding each cell like a balloon. As you exhale, imagine letting the balloons completely deflate and blow any tension or toxins that remain in the body out into the air. Continue doing this slowly for a few minutes, watching the balloons expand and contract.

Healing Image

Imagine little workers repairing the muscles and bones while they are resting, allowing the healing process to begin. See the bone rich in calcium, and see little bone cells growing like coral, increasing in number and density.

Ideal Images

Many clients continue to envision their healing processes long after the crises have passed. One way they do this is to imagine themselves in three or six months. They can imagine themselves exactly as they would wish to be. They can observe how they look, how they walk, their facial expressions. They might imagine themselves running or swimming, looking healthy and happy.

It is also a good practice for nurses to see themselves as they want to be. Focus on the image; how does it feel to be whole? Many nurses find that using imagery supports their patients totally and empowers them in their work. According to one nurse, after incorporating imagery frequently, "I finally felt as if I were making a difference, despite the disempowering aspects of the environment."

DEALING WITH FEAR AND ANXIETY

One of the three nurses mentioned in connection with the imagery workshop, Susan Ezra, works in her private practice part-time, and part-time at Hospice with oncology and AIDS patients. She also offers some very helpful advice that is especially designed to alleviate anxiety for nurses interested in using imagery in their work.

Tapes for Patients

Susan suggests that nurses interested in therapeutic imagery begin to research the tapes on the subject. In this process, the nurse can utilize the tapes that inspire her while working with her clients. She feels it is helpful for nurses to begin to make these tapes available for our clients.

She advises nurses to consider pooling their resources and starting a tape library where patients can be introduced in their own timing to this powerful healing tool. The equipment needed for this endeavor is minimal—merely a cassette recorder that allows for personal use.

Working with the Breath

Susan has a strong background in yoga, and feels it is important to work with the breath. She feels that we do this in labor and delivery, and perhaps have a tendency to neglect the potential for using breath consciously in many other medical situations. According to Susan, sometimes it is enough to merely encourage the patient to breathe into the belly and relax. This simple exercise provides a whole body relaxation.

Counting with the Breath

Susan also reminds us of one of the simpler methods to encourage revitalization; counting backward from 10 to 1. This exercise is coupled with breathing; a slow breath is taken and upon the exhale, the client says the number to himself, or aloud. A suggestion is given beforehand that when the client reaches 1, he will be recharged and relieved.

The guide frequently needs to encourage people to slow their breathing. Simple slow deep breathing activates the relaxation response.

Working with Fear

Breathing is a powerful physiological process. Many ancient traditions, including yoga, work with the breath to encourage energy flow. Energy can become blocked in numerous places in the body. Breathing can increase the energy flow and help to remove any blockages.

Working with the breath is working with energy, or life force. When one is focused on breathing, there is an inward experience, a meditative state is induced. There can also be a powerful release of blocked energy in a variety of forms. Breathing can be transformative, and many ancient and modern therapies focus solely or in large part on the breath.

SUMMARY

There are a great many ways to begin to work with imagery in nursing. The next section will review the process for finding one's special place, then it will explore further how the nurse can help the client access the inner guide and use the inner guide for basic healing maneuvers.

References

Acterberg, J., Dossey, B., & Kolkmeier, L. (1994). *Rituals of healing: Using imagery for health and wellness.* New York: Bantam Books.

Benson, H. (1984). *Beyond the relaxation response.* New York: Times Books.

Gershon, D., & Straub, G. (1989). *Empowerment: The art of creating your life as you want it.* New York: Dell Publishing.

Nightingale, F. (1859). *Notes on nursing.* London: Churchill Livingstone.

Rossman, M., & Bresler, D. (1982). *Introductory literature: Academy of guided imagery.* Mill Valley, CA: Academy of Guided Imagery.

Simonton, O.C., & Matthews-Simonton, S. (1978). *Getting well again.* Los Angeles: J.P. Tarcher.

C h a p t e r

5

INTERMEDIATE CLINICAL APPLICATIONS: INDIVIDUALIZING IMAGERY EXPERIENCES

If we allow ourselves to enter the quiet, still place of prayerfulness, we can understand the co-relationship of health and illness in the natural order.

Larry Dossey, MD, 1993

Once the client has successfully accomplished the initial steps of relaxation and has found a special place (either of which is enough for a basic introductory experience), the practitioner may wish to proceed with the process of helping the client find an inner guide. (Note: the term *inner guide* will be used for the balance of this book to refer to what the Academy for Guided Imagery calls the *inner advisor.*) In the next section, we will review inner guide concepts prior to advancing to more sophisticated techniques.

REVIEW: MEETING THE INNER GUIDE

Keep in mind that meeting the inner guide can happen very quickly for some people and be very elusive for others. There is no one right way for this process to occur, nor is it a necessity. Many clients receive tremendous benefit from simply relaxing and knowing that they have a safe place to go to whenever they want.

87

It is also important to remember, however, that meeting the inner guide is an excellent way of accessing inner wisdom. It can be a wonderful and powerful experience to help people connect with their own inner resources. Although we all have inner resources, we often forget to use them, especially when we are in crisis.

Introducing the Inner Guide

There are other reasons to help people meet their inner guides. First, it provides inner acceptance and self-love. Next, it allows deeper exploration of a problem, symptom, or conflict. Third, people can use their inner wisdom to mediate between the various parts of themselves (for instance, the part that wishes to get well versus the part that enjoys the dependency position). It also allows people a way to explore unresolved issues. Mostly, this process encourages clients to connect with their own truths.

Likewise, there are benefits with continued use of this process. It allows people to develop a relationship with themselves. It encourages them to feel good about just *being*, rather than always having to do something. It enhances communication, giving a firm sense of knowingness.

For some people, the inner guide process provides a new friend; it creates a relationship that is trustworthy, valuable, and ongoing. Keep in mind that for some people, meeting the inner guide can be a very emotional experience. It may be the first time they have connected with such love or support.

Most of all, however, the focus or intent of this work is on the *experience*. For many clients, the use of imagery provides a positive and healing experience.

General Guidelines for Inner Guide Work

Keep in mind, as discussed in the previous section, that imagery allows a person a positive and helpful experience. To ensure that this is so, there are several things to keep in mind. First, when leading a person in the inner guidance process, pay attention visually and intuitively. Watch his eye movements, facial expressions, and breathing. Many practitioners find that it is helpful to pace their breathing to the breath of the client. In that way, the two merge into a unified team, working collaboratively. This also sends a subtle message to the client that he is in charge and does not have to feel rushed or pressured.

You might recall that in chapter 4 the concept of the inner advisor (guide) was discussed in greater detail. It was stated then that this idea will be perceived differently by every person. Some people see the inner guide as a Higher Power, God or Goddess, Great Spirit, or whatever their traditions offer.

As previously mentioned, the qualities of the inner guide include unconditional love, nonjudgmental attitude, honesty, wisdom, compassion, patience, and optimism. The inner guide is usually contacted once the client has achieved a comfortable state of relaxation, and at times after the client has found a safe place.

The client can then invite an image of his inner guide to be with him. Rather than actively imagine that entity, he can be encouraged to allow an image to form, one that represents a wise, loving part of himself. It does not matter whether the image comes in a human or animal form, or even a sensation, as long as it feels loving.

The following script is supplied by Terry Miller, RN, MS, as an example of introduction.

Sample Imagery Script: Finding One's Special Place

Begin by placing your body in a comfortable position, arms and legs uncrossed, back well supported. Now take three deep breaths, allowing each breath to relax you even more. Let the exhalation be a letting go kind of breath, letting go of tension. With each in breath, take in what you need and with each out breath, release anything you don't need. Bring your attention to the top of your head. Feel your scalp relax and let your brow soften and smooth out. Allow all the little muscles around your eyes to relax. And let any tension flow out through your cheeks as you exhale. Suggest that your jaw relax.

Imagine a wave of relaxation flowing down your shoulders, into your arms, elbows, forearms, all the way into your hands and fingers. Now focus on your chest, releasing any tension around your heart or lungs, relax the muscles around your ribs. Wrap that relaxation around your back and let a wave of relaxation travel all down the spine. Allow the muscles along the spine to lengthen and release. Soften and relax the buttocks and pelvis. Let the belly be very soft so that the breath moves easily down into the abdomen. Invite the legs to join in the relaxation now, as it moves through the thighs, knees, calves, ankles, and feet. Let any last bit of tension or tightness just drain out through your feet and toes. When you feel relaxed and comfortable, let me know with a nod of your head. As your body remains relaxed and comfortable, imagine yourself in a very special place, somewhere that is full of natural beauty, safety, and peace. It may be a place you have been to before or it may be a place you want to create in your imagination. Take some time and let yourself be drawn to one place that is just right for you today. Let me know when you are present there (wait for response). Describe what it is like there. What do you see? Are there any smells? Are there any sounds? What is the temperature like? Where are you in this special place? How do you feel here? Take some time to do whatever you would like to do here, to relax or do some activity. Feel free to do whatever you want. This is your place.

In a few moments, it will be time to come back into a waking state. Know that you can return to this place again any time you want. Now gently bring yourself back, letting the images fade but keeping with you this relaxed and peaceful feeling. Remember what has been important about this experience. Become aware of the current time and place. Begin to move your body, take a deep breath, open your eyes, and feel relaxed and awake.

At this point, the guide can take a few minutes to allow the person to share his experience.

This is one example of an introductory experience to find one's special place. There are many variations that can deepen and enrich the relaxation. In some instances, after finding his special place, the client can be encouraged to meet someone in his special place and to talk with the guide who appears.

The client can then be encouraged to ask questions of the inner guide, then listen to any response (as was presented in the earlier session with Suzanne). This contact alone can have a dramatic impact on the client.

Considerations When Accessing Inner Guide

Keep in mind that big issues can arise around trust. Some people are extremely cautious, perhaps afraid of facing certain thoughts or aspects of themselves. These people may want some assurance that they will not encounter a situation that they feel unable to handle.

For these reasons, it is always safer to ask the client about his beliefs, rather than to assume anything. As an example, consider the client being guided through a visualization experience. The practitioner, intending to be helpful and provide a relaxing image, suggests that the client close his eyes and imagine himself at the beach. He is instructed to watch the ocean waves roll in and out, hypnotically inducing a state of relaxation.

For many people, this is an extremely effective image for relaxation. However, for the person who has never been to the beach (yes, they do exist!), or for someone who has a fear of the ocean, this image does anything *but* support relaxation. A striking example of someone who may not fare well with this image is a person who had a relative drown or who almost drowned as a child. If a person saw a ship go down or lost a friend in the stormy seas, or even in a pool, this image may evoke terrifying memories.

Another often-used example is provided by the practitioner who suggests that the client close his eyes and picture himself riding an elevator from the top floor down to the basement, perhaps even visualizing the numbers as they would look from inside the elevator going down during the descent. This is a powerful method for bringing a person into a highly relaxed state of mind, but it has been known to backfire more than once. One reason for this is that many people do not like to ride elevators; some are even claustrophobic. For these people, the image is not a friendly, relaxing one. Examples such as these help us to validate the special gifts of interactive imagery, when the client supplies the images.

For these reasons, the practitioner must be very aware of helping the client who doesn't feel completely safe. The client can be encouraged to create a special place in his mind, and use the imagination in a variety of ways to enhance a sense of personal safety. The practitioner can also go slowly, pacing according to the client's response.

Building trust is an integral component of the process. The practitioner can build upon the client's previous successes, help to solidify the state of relaxation, and take time to educate the client thoroughly prior to working in this manner. The client can also be encouraged to surround himself with a protective bubble; if necessary, it can even be located in the sky where no one can reach it or invade it. The mind is endless in its creative potential.

Guiding Clients Through Emotional Experiences

It is important to keep in mind that some people become very emotional when meeting an inner advisor. There are several reasons for this. First, the form of the advisor may represent someone they know and love or have known and loved. This happened to the author in a large audience while being invited to meet my inner guide. I quickly recognized the form of my dear departed grandmother, who had been a tremendous source of strength and inspiration to me in earlier years. When I saw her, I burst out crying loudly, and I was surprised by my own response. This sort of emotional release can be part of the healing that is needed, even when we don't know that. The therapist or guide should always be sure to allow time to deal with unexpected outbursts.

It can also be very emotional to meet the inner guide in that it is like reconnecting with a lost part of one's self. In this relaxed, safe place, feelings can be easily aroused, and the guide needs to be prepared to handle emotionality. If the nurse is not trained well in psychiatry or does not feel comfortable, she may wish to advance her knowledge base or comfort level prior to using advanced techniques.

Suggestions for Practitioners

Keep in mind that as a guide, you don't have to *do* anything; you don't have to "fix it." One of the aspects of this work that makes it so appealing, as distinguished from psychotherapy, is that there is no "rescue" expected. The client is the one setting the pace for the experience. He can choose to do nothing, to leave the mental creation, to back up, or even to call upon his inner guide to hold his hand if need be. This is a very creative process, and the client is empowered to make the best decisions for himself.

Advancing Your Skills As Practitioner

Inner guide work can be very deep. People who would like to use this type of process frequently want to extend their knowledge bases for more in-depth work. Please refer to the Resource Guide in the Appendix, and especially to the Academy for Guided Imagery in Mill Valley, CA for further study.

INTERMEDIATE IMAGERY IN THE CLINICAL SETTING

We will now explore the ways in which the nurse can make a difference in the clinical setting using more advanced imagery techniques. Keep in mind that continuing in any one imagery process is always a matter of the client's choice, and that clients can proceed or not according to their inner pace and feelings.

A Simple Example

In the workshop called "Beyond Ordinary Nursing," Susan Ezra, RN, Jan Maxwell, RN, BA, and Terry Miller, RN, MS, gave this anecdote to remind prospective guides that clients always have a choice. They talked about a radio show that was popular when they were young that featured Bill Cosby, a well-known comedian. One of his most famous routines was about a chicken heart that was loudly beating and pounding as it ascended the stairs (seemingly toward the listener). The pounding became louder and louder and Cosby was yelling above the sound, as if terrified. This image did, in fact, terrify young members of his radio audience. It was so memorable that many in our imagery class were able to recall seeing that image years ago in their mind's eye.

The three instructors then asked us how many of us had thought, as a child, of jumping up and turning the knob on the radio so we would no longer be tormented. A surprising number of people had not thought of that. We were reminded that in imagery work, the images can seem as loud and frightening as this chicken heart thundering up the stairs.

Another memorable example comes from Dr. Seuss's "Glunk that got thunk" image. A young girl would use her "thinker-upper" to amuse herself, and she thought up an image that was annoying. Finally, her brother came in; together they "unthunk the glunk."

We can always exercise the choice to switch our thoughts to a more pleasant and comfortable image, or even imagine turning the image off. When we are working with images which are total mental constructs we are in the position to direct the scene creatively.

Advice for Beginning Nurses Using Imagery

It is crucial to keep in mind that *more* is not always better. Doing relaxation exercises and finding a special place can be enough. For many of our clients, this is a tremendous gift, as they may be so laden with fear and anxiety that they can not find a safe place by themselves.

This is especially true for people who were abused in childhood. For these individuals, there was never a place that felt safe, and they learned to live in constant terror that their boundaries would be invaded.

It is also advisable to remember that using guided imagery is *not* recommended with patients who are identified as having a psychotic or schizophrenic process or history. It is generally considered that these people are often bombarded with too many images already, and are unable to differentiate between those they choose to envision and those that plague their mental processes involuntarily. The use of imagery requires an ability to sustain one's focus and concentration. These patients are usually not able to maintain these components.

The guide holds the space for the client to feel safe. As we create a healing environment, the client gradually acquires a sense of control and peacefulness. When we are calm and centered, our intent is focused on the expansion of the person's sense of security, we give the client permission to relax.

How to Make Time for Imagery

Most nurses feel so overwhelmed that they are reluctant to entertain the thought of trying to squeeze any more activities into their schedules. They tend to think of adding imagery as one more chore to be done.

Quite the contrary, when a nurse makes time for relaxation or imagery in her busy day, she is giving both herself and her client a great gift. The time alone makes clients feel cared for, and special. The process supports a relaxation of the muscles and an easing of tensions and fear, even if only for a short while. It is certain that this state allows for a greater absorption of pharmaceuticals as well as other treatments.

Most nurses who give special moments of caring to their patients find that the patients are less demanding and needy, and more cooperative. In the long run, the nurse often saves herself time by giving special attention early on in the process.

An equally wonderful gift, however, is the one the nurse provides for herself when she takes a few minutes of special caring with her clients. In those small moments and gestures, the nurse reconnects with her heart, her spirit, her desire to be part of the healing process. When a nurse takes special time, centers herself, and offers relaxation, she is rewarded. No longer is she just another part of the machinery, endlessly ticking away until she wears out. She is now rejuvenating herself in those quiet moments, reminding herself to stay connected to all that nursing means to her and to all that she has to offer through this labor of love. In this sense, imagery offers a win-win scenario.

Developing Open-Mindedness

To be nurses who do imagery work effectively, we must be open-minded and prepared to honor a great variety of belief systems in our work. There is no room in healing work for prejudice or judgments about people who are different.

As nurses, we have to let go of our assumptions and expectations. We may have our own ideas about how we prefer to be treated, but advancing our ideas is not our role. The nurse is not there to direct the outcome.

This way of thinking might be very different for many nurses, for we have been trained under a much more domineering model. Nonetheless, nursing is progressing as an art and science that is unique in many ways, and one that is destined to develop further compassion and tolerance.

Imagery provides a person with the opportunity to realize his dreams, find his empowerment or success, come to grips with whatever it is that he needs, give in to the process, and learn to surrender. All of these components are part of the healing journey.

Examples of Making Time

Terry Miller, RN, MS, frequently used imagery when she worked in the Intensive Care Unit. She regularly noted the beneficial results of taking time for imagery. When she did relaxation with her patients on nipride drips, she found that she had to quickly decrease the drips and frequently turn them off, actually using less of the medication.

Terry found that medical-surgical nursing units can be very challenging places to use imagery, in large part because of the issue of time in nurse-patient ratios. As she became more comfortable and proficient, she learned to approach the client early in the shift. If the client was anxious or in pain, she would ask him "Would you like to learn how to relax?" She found that not many patients would say "no."

Terry found that she could plan her day around an imagery session. She also learned to take risks to allow for the maximum benefit. Often, for example, she placed a sign on the door when in session (with the client's permission) that read "Do not disturb for 5 minutes." This created a safe, sometimes sacred, space in which Terry and her client could work together uninterrupted.

She also found that sessions could be done very simply and informally. An example of this is when she took a few minutes to sit next to a client and encouraged him to take a few deep breaths.

As a word of encouragement to nurses trying to make time for relaxation, Terry suggests taking very small steps. As you notice a small window of opportunity, take it and experiment with it until you devise your own systems. Keep in mind that as you support the relaxation of your clients, you get to experience it as well.

Legal Considerations

Nurses often wonder whether they need specific orders to use imagery or other healing tools when they are beginning to incorporate these tools into their practices. No order is needed because providing comfort measures and helping patients cope is a large part of nursing practice. Some nurses chart "*therapeutic relaxation*" when providing a session. Others consider providing comfort merely another aspect of good bedside manner and patient care.

We have seen that imagery and relaxation are particularly helpful when used immediately prior to a painful procedure or time, and are best when used before the pain mounts. Nurses often note that patients are weaned from drips sooner and require less medication when relaxation exercises are provided early. All of these observations may be documented accordingly.

Some nurses take machine printouts and mark when imagery was done, often demonstrating a significant clinical change immediately post-relaxation. This is a valuable method for enticing other nurses and health professionals to consider the benefits of this work.

The California Nurses Association (1982) issued a position statement on relaxation. It states "It is the interpretation of the CNA that a Registered Nurse who is adequately prepared with verified education and experience in these therapies is practicing within the bounds of the Nurse Practice Act."

Nurse practice acts vary from state to state. The California Nurse Practice Act specifies that nurses are expected to help their patients cope with different health situations. Nursing practice aims to help people cope with difficulties in daily living that are associated with their actual or potential health or illness problems, or treatment, which requires a substantial amount of scientific knowledge or technical skill. This direct and indirect service ensures safety, comfort, personal hygiene, and protection of patients, and the performance of disease prevention and restorative measures.

We can see that according to the definition of nursing as presented in the California Nurse Practice Act, gentle relaxation tools are very much considered to be an essential part of our nursing work.

An Example: What Nurses Do

In one moving example, a nurse was at the bedside of a dying patient. The doctor saw the nurse as she was sitting beside the patient, breathing gently in unison with the person. The two appeared to be so supportively connected that the doctor turned to a nearby nurse and said "I didn't know Susie has a relative in the ICU." The nurse turned to him and said, "No, doctor, that's not her relative. That's a part of what nurses do!"

Creative Nursing

In another example, a nurse was working with an agitated dying patient who had always wanted to go to Europe. It was apparent that the wish would never be fulfilled. The nurse took ten minutes of relaxation in a quiet place with the patient, mentally escorting him to a quiet place where he felt comfortable and had no pain. The nurse gently guided the patient by asking questions such as "Where would you like to go?"; "What would you like to do?"; and "How does that feel?" When she looked over, the patient was crying and said he really felt that he had gone to Europe, and that it was wonderful. Within two days the patient died very peacefully.

OTHER USES OF IMAGERY

Several nurses report very positive results using relaxation and imagery prior to, during, and after procedures such as intubation, cardiac catheterization, and chemotherapy. Likewise, these tools are known to be quite helpful when dealing with same-day surgery experiences.

An example of this is a breast biopsy, where the woman undergoes surgery and does not know the results. In this case, the client often feels very out of control. When asked where she would like to go to create a safe space, she might say "the mountains" or "the ocean." At these times, it can be helpful to invite her to create an affirmation while in her favorite natural setting.

BIRTH-RELATED IMAGERY

There are many opportunities to introduce imagery to women who are involved in the childbirth process. We will now explore some of these times when imagery can be helpful.

Antepartum

For women who are hospitalized awaiting complicated childbirths and for those who are admitted to be monitored, the endless sitting in a hospital bed can produce boredom. These women can become quite irritable and may be internally pressured by their inability to function. They may have left children and loved ones at home, and feel concerned or guilty as a result, or they may have left work unfinished in their professional lives. They may bemoan their lost wages. For these patients, a visit to a sacred space might be exactly the medicine that is needed.

Many obstetrical nurses encourage their patients to envision their babies, and to make contact with them on some level. To do this, the woman must feel relaxed, safe, and supported. Often, pregnant women enjoy creating and building connections and loving relationships with the baby in utero. When the fetus is very small, women sometimes enjoy imagining what it will look like when it is larger.

Labor Imagery

There are countless ways women can be supported using imagery during childbirth. Though we cannot discuss all of them here, some practical examples are included to inspire the nurse to create opportunities to use this powerful tool for birthing.

Midwives and nurses in delivery situations have reported positive results from encouraging a mother with a breech to imagine the baby turning his head down to deliver safely. Women in labor often imagine the mighty contractions as natural cycles of the ocean. Some see an image of a lotus flower opening.

Family and friends can do visualizations during a birth, whether or not they are present in the labor room. Recent research has demonstrated that sending loving thoughts, or non-local prayer, has an effect across time and space (Dossey, 1993).

Postpartum Imagery

Nurses working with women postpartum also find imagery a powerful adjunct to nursing care. The new mother has many special challenges at this time, including viewing herself as a mother if this is her first child. She also has to cope with changes in the dynamics of her marriage if she is married, and major changes in her lifestyle under all circumstances. If there are other children, the woman has to integrate the new family member. She must cope with major hormonal shifts and financial pressures. Imagery can be useful to initiate breastfeeding.

Imagery can be extremely helpful for the new mother, whether it is offered immediately postpartum or at home or during clinic visits. This tool can be shared with a woman early in the pregnancy, and it may be something she learns to use in stressful times for the rest of her life. This tool can be instrumental in teaching parents new coping skills for their expanded roles. Children are also very receptive to using imagery to cope with separations and frightening procedures.

In fact, teaching new parents to find a safe, restful place may eventually impact the child and spousal abuse statistics. Nurses are in a perfect strategic position to start making a difference in some social conditions, for we work with people in crises and can teach them healthy new skills.

AFFIRMATIONS AND IMAGERY

An *affirmation* has been described as a positive statement that affirms an experience one wishes. It has also been described as a nutrient for the soul. Affirmations are closely related to what has often been called wishful thinking. The statement is frequently based on some perception of need ("I am a strong and vibrant person") in which the most positive outcome is affirmed ("I will feel wonderful during this procedure, and the biopsy will be negative").

Affirmations can be woven into imagery in many creative ways. An example of this would be to have the client envision a healing and powerful scene, then take the information received in the imagery experience and create an affirmation to use regularly afterwards. For example, if a client uses imagery to access an inner guide, then comes out of the relaxed state with a name and feeling of his guide, he might affirm, "I feel loved and supported in the presence of Maya" (his guide). He can continue to affirm Maya's love and support in his daily existence. He might even be encouraged to feel Maya's love filling his heart, then carry that feeling with him into his daily life.

At times, when a client is encouraged to pursue a particular statement that has great emotional charge, he will meet with enormous feelings. One person, who never felt loved when growing up, chose as an affirmation "I am lovable." As he repeated this statement, he would feel a tremendous emotional release. After many months of working with this affirmation, the client had released the charge on the words, and he was able to speak them and believe them. This was a very healing process for him.

Affirming Good Health: Creative Uses

Another poignant example was provided several years ago at a nursing conference. A physician was reporting on her work with women, and told the audience that she had supported a friend of hers recently who had asked her to be involved in her first surgical experience. The friend was frightened and asked the doctor, who was a psychiatrist, if she would be her advocate during surgery. The patient firmly believed that she would be aware of everything that was said and done during the procedure, and had heard stories about the callous joke-telling episodes that often occur in the operating room. The patient asked her doctor-friend to tell the other doctors that the patient felt very strongly about what might transpire in the operating room while she was being operated on. The request was that any thoughts or statements be totally positive and affirming of a healthy outcome. Needless to say, the OR staff was surprised at such a request, but they were respectful of the woman's wishes. The surgery went extremely well, and the results were very positive. This is another example of affirming good health.

Nurses and health care team members can align themselves to support individual patients, provide continuity of care by sharing information about what has proved helpful and meaningful to the client, and thus reinforce consistency.

HABITS, ADDICTIONS, AND IMAGERY

Many of the motivational books and tapes currently available talk about habits and addictions. They remind us that people are indeed creatures of habit, and that we all operate a majority of the time on the habits we've acquired and developed.

According to the popular literature, we are either master of our habits or slave to them. These reference sources, vastly familiar to most of us in modern society, speak significantly about the problem of imbalance in habit, also known as addiction.

In the addictive process, the person attempts to fill some perceived hole in his life, often as a result of childhood deprivation of one sort or another. If you felt neglected or hurt by those you loved as a child, you might have grown up with a confusion between love and pain. Many of us in this culture have some lack of clarity regarding these major issues, and we seek relationships with people, processes, or substances in our attempts to numb the grief and sense of loss we feel.

In addictive behavior, we expend a great deal of energy looking outside ourselves for the answers to problems that lie within us. Not only do the problems lie within us, but the answers as well are available inside. In our desperate search to fill what we perceive as a hole inside, we look to other people, food, drugs, sexual encounters, and sometimes even dangerous behavior to fill that sense of longing and desperation.

Addictive Thinking: Overcoming Negative Patterns

People also become addicted to certain patterns of thinking which may have been taught to them or which may have served their needs in earlier times. They cling tenaciously to patterns that actually limit their freedom and capacity to act in their own best interests. When this occurs, sickness invariably ensues.

As an example, consider the person who has three glasses of milk daily, as had always been recommended by the dietary industry in our country. That person, over the years, has developed chronic constipation and excess flatulence, to the point of frequently being unable to perform normal duties.

A visit to a holistically oriented physician informs the client that he could be dealing with a stress-related allergic disorder. To evaluate the problem, it is suggested that the client list everything eaten for a three-day period.

When the physician and client jointly review the diet history, it becomes obvious that the client consumes a lot of one item, milk. The physician proposes that the client experiment by eliminating that item from the diet temporarily to see what effect that change might have. The client becomes enraged.

"That's the most ridiculous thing I've ever heard," he mutters. "I've been drinking three glasses of milk a day for my entire life. This problem only started a few years ago. It can't be the milk!"

In this case, the client's refusal to review his habits may be detrimental to his health. He has adopted a rather rigid viewpoint, one that does not make room for new ideas or allow for creativity.

As previously stated, habits can be our allies or enemies. Keeping our minds habitually closed to new possibilities is one way we allow ourselves to remain stuck in ruts. Tenacious, stubborn patterns of thinking prevent collective progress, and in the individual person, can prevent healing. The hold these thoughts have over us is not to be underestimated.

The creation of new affirmations, along with open-minded exploration and willingness to change, can transform a situation that has been ruled by negative thinking into a positive, life-affirming one. The choice is ours.

Working with Unhealthy Habits

One of the easiest and simplest maneuvers is to imagine a new habit replacing an old one. For example, in considering the client who had been told he was allergic to milk, the client could imagine drinking three cups of herbal tea a day instead of the milk. He could, in his imagery, see himself feeling better and having his symptoms relieved. Rather than being incapacitated, he moves forward in his productivity with a renewed sense of clarity and purpose. As the imagery becomes more clear and solid in his mind, the transition in his real life, from milk to herbal tea, is facilitated. His ability to picture himself making this change readily eases the process.

A more advanced technique for the client, if it had been needed, might have involved using imagery to go back in his memory and re-experience the origin of the milk habit. He might have seen that his habit was largely due to the urgings of a kindly nanny who made the milk a gesture of closeness and kindness. He might now use his imagery to create other ways to provide himself with warmth and relaxation, rather than with this ill-advised substance.

Imagery and the Addiction Process

Likewise, imagery can be helpful for a number of even more harmful habits, including alcohol abuse. Recovery practitioners have long known that part of the stubbornness of this harmful habit is related to two major imagery factors.

First, the alcoholic has developed a keen ability to easily envision himself having a drink whenever the going gets tough. In addition, the alcoholic lacks the training to creatively envision himself choosing a healthier option. In other words, he sees himself having a drink instead of seeing himself saying "no" to the drink and doing something else.

When imagery is used to give the alcoholic the novel idea that there are nonalcoholic options that will work better, there is a much greater chance that his life choices will follow. A person trained in imagery begins to envision himself calling his sponsor when the going gets tough or attending more meetings for added support. At some point, the person relies less and less on external resources and learns more and more about utilizing his inner guidance and resources.

This is a fine example of how imagery assists people in making more powerful choices related to their own sense of well-being. In this manner, imagery inspires a deep level of healing to occur.

IMAGERY IN ONCOLOGY

Cancer might well be the most feared disease of our times. Many people live their lives in dread and fear of cancer. The traditional medical treatments are terrifying and excruciating. Many nurses find it beneficial to work with the client's negative images and beliefs.

Some nurses have reported making tapes (there are also some available commercially) in which the client is encouraged to imagine chemotherapy or radiation therapy as something positive. Some clients prefer to view it as beams of energy or light.

The practitioner might ask "How do you imagine the chemotherapy?" Despite the response, the nurse can be helpful in supporting the transformation of the images into something beneficial and positive. "Imagine the medicine going into exactly the cells that most need it. The side effects will be minimal." There are a great variety of techniques and applications that enhance the healing journey through the experience of cancer. In chapter 7, a beautiful example is provided of a nurse who was diagnosed with cancer and used imagery to help herself heal.

Simonton Technique

O. Carl Simonton and Stephanie Matthews-Simonton performed groundbreaking work using creative visualization with oncology patients. In their work, they taught patients to visualize strong, healthy immune system cells fighting against the cancer cells.

It is felt that this work can be useful for many chronic challenges, and, in that sense, visualization and imagery have a special role with people for whom the medical system has little to offer. In those instances, this tool can be a last hope. It is certainly a less costly and less invasive maneuver and is therefore worthy of serious consideration.

The Simonton technique gives clients the chance to try to affect what is happening in their bodies. Once again, it is not crucial that every image be anatomically correct. What is important is that the client is assertive and has a chance to be effective.

Though many of the Simonton clients worked with aggressive battlelike images, this is not the only way to use this technique. The client may wish to affirm: "My cells and my intelligence will be mobilized to fight this disease off."

Remember, the images can be realistic or metaphorical. One creative client invented a machine that was constantly producing millions of white blood cells. Another client had white knights and black knights doing battle (the leader of the white knights was Joan of Arc). Others imagine fish (immune system cells) swimming through the vessels, finding the cancer cells, eating them, then digesting and destroying them.

Other images include cats, wolves, or dogs devouring abnormal cells, and birds eating the seeds of cancer. It is helpful for the client to have a guide in cases of frightening images. The guide can ask "What would you like to have happen?", then she can encourage the client to bring the image to that scenario. Remember that we have to be careful of our assumptions and give the client opportunities to take control. We can remind him that it is his image.

A Positive Example

One nurse shared the case of an oncologist she worked with. In this situation, the tables were turned, and the doctor was the nurse's patient. The doctor had had surgery recently for prostate cancer and was seeking new ways to cope with his ongoing fear of recurrence. It was, in the nurse's words, "an honor to be his guide."

Through this life crisis, the doctor explored his power and spirit, reclaiming his soul. He imagined forest, trees, and waterfalls, and was able to contact his power animal. (According to Native-American tradition, all people have animal guides walking beside them in their lives to offer wisdom and protection; these people believe that one reason so many Caucasian people are ill is that they don't properly utilize their power animals.)

This oncologist-patient seemed to have made the decision to use his disease to develop his inner resources. As he so eloquently stated, "Healing has to come from the magic within."

Imagery Rehearsal

Once a little-known concept, today imagery rehearsal is used in many arenas. Sports trainers are incorporating this tool to inspire peak performance in athletes. The process is a very supportive one. It builds hope, allows a person to see himself with an ideal self-image, and enables him to imagine a positive outcome. In working with cancer patients, the guide might suggest, "Imagine yourself feeling/being/looking exactly the way you want to be."

The nurse can use imagery rehearsal to decrease fear or to assuage nausea and vomiting in oncology patients. Nurses report that imagery helps with anticipatory nausea (when some cancer patients remember the last chemotherapy experience and psychologically induce a state of nausea prior to treatment). This technique also helps with cumulative nausea.

The client can be encouraged to imagine the antinausea drugs given during his treatment as the drugs go to the brain and are properly dispersed to the body before, during, and after the treatment. Nausea can be difficult to directly influence, yet many advantageous results have been demonstrated after positive rehearsal for the accompanying fatigue and hair loss.

SUGGESTED IMAGERY TECHNIQUES FOR PAIN

In this section, we will further explore specific techniques that are helpful in working naturally with people in pain.

Breathing

We have mentioned the importance of breathing in previous sections of this chapter. There are some simple ways to work with people in pain using the breath.

Encourage the client to take a deep inward breath and release it. Then have the client proceed to the next inhalation. Have him breathe into that painful part, using the breath to release the pain. Help the client relax between the breaths.

Many women have found the following technique lifesaving while giving birth naturally. It is also useful for dealing with other kinds of cyclic pain, such as intestinal spasms. Have the client take quick shallow breaths as a wave of pain reaches its crescendo, moving into slower, deeper cleansing breaths between the waves of pain.

Working with the Image of the Pain

Ask the client to describe the pain. Have him be as descriptive as possible ("It's like a sharp knife sticking between my ribs"). Then ask him how he feels about it ("I hate it; it's killing me"). Then ask him what he wants, and have him envision that.

A person with metastatic cancer had an image of a bright red burning ball. The nurse asked him what was in the ball. The client said there was anger in the ball: anger at the cancer and at some people in his life. The guide worked with these images. She asked "What do you want to do with the ball?" The client responded that he wanted to throw it into the ocean, as far as he could, and to watch it sink. By actively creating this vision, his pain was significantly reduced.

Another example is a nurse who had a severe, sudden onset of neck pain. The pain was excruciating and radiated down her arm (diagnosis was herniated neck disk). The client had an image of a big rusty machine that needed to be polished. It changed forms. Through diligent work with imagery and other gentle healing techniques, including physical therapy, the disk gradually resolved.

One exercise that can be helpful is to bring an image of fear to mind. The client can likewise bring images of comfort or pain to mind. In guided imagery, the visions supplied are usually positive ones provided by the practitioner. In interactive imagery, on the other hand, the practitioner helps the client to work with whatever images arise.

In these situations, the images are occasionally scary. It is known in psychological work that fears seem to grow if they are not addressed. On the other hand, when we face the fears, they often seem not so scary, and they tend to dissipate.

Work with the image can be accomplished in a variety of ways. The practitioner can have the client continue to see the image and observe how it changes under varying conditions. The client can be encouraged to dialogue with the image or to envision different interventions and their effects on the image. This is a more advanced technique, and should generally be done by someone who has had extended imagery training. It is often best accomplished by practitioners with advanced psychotherapy training as well.

There is a technique to work with the image of pain in three stages. First, the patient works with the image at its worst. The practitioner can suggest that the patient imagine the pain when it's been at its worst. (It is better to do this process when the patient is not in severe pain.) Have the patient spend time observing and understanding the image that arises. Now move to the image of the pain at its best. Help the patient to pace forward to an image when the pain is gone, or when relief is felt. Remember to use the patient's words.

Susan Ezra gives us another example. She had a bout with eczema on her right hand (often considered to be the side related to giving). She recalled the image at its worst; the image was very red, inflamed, and painful. She then recalled the image at its best, where it was much less red and inflamed. The third time Susan saw the image, it was not a hand at all, but instead was her as a whole person. The focus of the image was not on her hand.

She also shares with us the story of an anesthesiologist who has AIDS and who was experiencing severe abdominal pain. In the first image, he saw a burning building, and he knew that it needed to burn itself out. In the second image, he was in a swimming pool, enjoying the sensation of floating on a raft. His third image had him walking his dog, feeling active and great.

Once you show a client this technique, he can practice it on his own. He can be encouraged to practice going from the worst to the best images, then into imagery rehearsal, and hopefully into total freedom from pain.

Glove Anesthesia Technique

There is also a slightly more advanced tool that can be useful for people experiencing pain unrelieved by other methods. Glove anesthesia is a classic hypnosis technique.

The patient is encouraged to relax and to feel that his hand is anesthetized. The practitioner might suggest that the patient has just stuck his hand in a big vat of anesthesia or snow, thus making it very numb. The patient then mentally transfers the anesthesia to painful areas as he touches them.

This is an example of a session that must be highly directed, usually by a well-trained practitioner. It is presented to demonstrate how we nurses can take the knowledge we have acquired about hypnosis and imagery and begin to expand the ideas into creative and meaningful solutions to unique and difficult problems.

WHERE TO START

To initiate these processes, the nurse can simply assist clients in becoming aware of any images they might have. She might start by talking with the clients about their conscious images of pain. She can have the clients draw their images, then see their pain when it is at its worst and best and when it is absent. The nurse will most enjoy adding this tool when she is able to creatively inspire the client to view his illness from a new perspective. There are a number of ways to assist the client in gaining a different view of his symptoms.

Intensity Scale

One easy-to-use tool is known as the intensity scale. This is a highly subjective tool that allows for some sense of comparison to emerge. The client can imagine an elevator dial or some other scale that is consecutively numbered from 1 to 10.

Ask the client to rate his degree of discomfort from 0 to 10 (where 0 represents no pain and 10 represents severe pain). If, for example, the client's answer is 6, the guide can suggest that the client deepen his state of relaxation by trying to see the dial go down from 6 to 5.

Continue working with the client on relaxing, breathing, and visualizing until he can get the number down as much as is likely during the time available. You might then suggest that the client lock the number there and thereby hold the pain at bay.

Once again, keep in mind that it is not always realistic for a client to be pain-free. Our goals for the client must be consistent with the client's goals for himself, and we must take care not to impose unrealistic expectations on him. If we are able to witness any evidence of improvement, comfort, or acceptance, we have helped.

Another useful technique, similar to the previous one, is to have the client visualize a thermometer rather than an elevator dial, and watch the numbers go up or down for the desired healing effect. In classic hypnosis, the client is frequently encouraged to make the pain worse and then better. In these processes, however, the client defines his own pain and gains a sense of mastery over it.

DIALOGUE WITH SYMPTOMS

Just as a client can learn to dialogue with his inner child, so can the client dialogue with a symptom. The client might view his noisy, destructive part as a childhood emotion stuck in time. Therefore, the symptom can be worked with as if it were a child requiring time and attention.

By directly confronting the symptom, and talking with it, the client often gains a deeper understanding of the meaning of the illness. Though it can be simple, this is actually a very powerful tool because the body seems to be quite sophisticated in its efforts to communicate with us.

CASE STUDY | *Laura*

Consider the case of a client who has herpes zoster, or shingles. This woman, Laura, had a recent episode of painful skin on her abdomen, which was not diagnosed medically. I was working with her to provide psychotherapy and disability counseling. She had a series of back problems and knew that many of her problems were psychological. She was referred to me for counseling by a very astute orthopedic physician who practices holistically.

Laura mentioned her painful abdominal skin in passing. She was puzzled and irritated by her condition, but was able to wear loose clothing and avoid too much discomfort. After several sessions, when Laura mentioned the discomfort casually, I encouraged her to make contact with the symptoms. She went to her inner place of safety, practiced progressive relaxation, then began to talk to the symptom. Some fascinating results ensued.

First, Laura got in touch with the part of herself that felt burned out and did not look forward to returning to any form of work. She felt exhausted and hopeful that she could find a way to complete her studies in psychology, rather than take menial jobs to support herself.

When she began to talk to the symptom, Laura had a startling realization: she saw that she had had this same symptom at an earlier time in her life. She had not remembered (until dialoguing with it) that when she was four years old, she had taken a long car trip with her grandparents. Her home life had been extremely chaotic, and she was aggrieved by the conditions in her immediate family.

On this trip, Laura recalled driving over many high bridges in the Northwest, and she was terrified. She eventually returned to her home and was hospitalized with a strange malady (after discovering that her parents had separated). The syndrome was never diagnosed to her knowledge, but the symptom was extremely painful skin across her abdomen that could not be touched.

Pattern Recognition

In recovering this memory, the client was able to recognize which parts of her current life resembled that earlier time. She realized that her strange symptoms appeared in her early life during a time of enormous upheaval and during circumstances that she perceived as frightening. Many years later, it seemed as if the same symptom reappeared during a time—you might have guessed—of great upheaval and fear. Though the exact circumstances were different, Laura was able to recognize patterns in her bodily response to certain types of stress.

According to Margaret Newman (1986), nursing theorist, this type of pattern recognition is extremely valuable in working with our clients. Laura was able to empower herself by noticing similar responses and by making decisions to change certain aspects of her life to alleviate the obvious stressors.

Had I, as her nurse-therapist, merely told her what I saw, she may not have gained the same connection to the material or had such a strong emotional reaction to her plight. Seeing it through her own eyes and sensing the information through this imagery process, Laura made wise decisions about her health on her own behalf. In this way, we can each become parent to our own wounded child inside. This is empowerment.

There are many other examples of pattern and symptom recognition that support the person's growth and well-being. Many authors claim to have developed systems for understanding the meaning of illness in various body parts. Many ancient cultures likewise embrace the philosophy that the body speaks, and we can learn to heal ourselves by listening to its symptoms.

Metaphors of Pain

If pain is the messenger, what is the message? Many practitioners enjoy encouraging clients to pay attention to their bodily symptoms and to imagine that each symptom has a voice. "What are the symptoms trying to tell you about your lifestyle?" This can be a playful, yet informative, method of healing.

For instance, it is often thought that the body can be viewed as a metaphor. Consider the saying "I can't stomach this" (particularly meaningful for stomach disorders). Another example is: "He's a royal pain in the neck."

Think about the many words that relate to the back, and how many back problems there are in our culture! *Back* related words include: *backed* against a wall, *backlash*, *back*-biting, *back*handed, and many others. When we are working with people with a particular illness, it can be fun and helpful to consider possible meanings in the illness.

IN THE FACE OF LOSS

Nursing is a natural place to share imagery work for other reasons as well. We nurses are the ones by the bedsides when people are severely ill or facing major losses in their lives. Whereas in the past we might have felt at a loss to know how to support the patient's journey, imagery now allows us to be with the people and their families in a unique and helpful manner.

CASE STUDY | *CEO Has Hip Replacement*

In her private practice, Terry Miller, RN, was fortunate to have the opportunity to work with a client six weeks prior to his hip surgery. Tony, being a "take charge" person, initiated the imagery sessions with clear objectives. He wanted to decrease his chronic pain (he had been a 9 on a pain-intensity scale of 1 to 10 for the past 2 1/2 years). He also wanted to prepare his body for surgery and to accelerate his healing and rehabilitation.

Relaxation and Inner Advisor

Terry first supported Tony in experiencing some progressive muscle relaxation and imaging in a safe, peaceful place. When Terry asked Tony to allow an image to appear that represented a part of him that was very wise and loving, a rabbi who was very sympathetic and willing to help Tony figure things out appeared. Tony's pain intensity decreased from 9 to 2 during this first session.

Grieving Work

Next, Tony was asked to allow an image to form that represented his hip joint. The image appeared bright red, swollen, and hot. In dialoguing with his hip, Tony obtained agreement from his hip that its time had come to an end. He told his hip how much he respected it and thanked it for doing its best for many years. When Tony asked his hip what it would advise, its reply was to make its sacrifice worthwhile, and Tony promised that he would.

Positive Rehearsal of Upcoming Surgery

The next session involved rehearsing the surgery as Tony wanted it to be. Top on Tony's list was to have his inner advisor, whom he called his protector, watch over the surgical team. He also wanted to work with his body to prevent complications. He imagined his immune system as hunters ("like cats stalking their prey"), and stationed those cats in the areas most likely to need protection. Tony saw the cats increase in number in those areas as if waiting in ambush, "ever ready to pounce on any foreign body."

The end of the session involved imaging the muscles and the area around the new hip preparing for new growth. Through the rehearsal session, Tony identified the need to have the surgeon talk to him during the surgery, letting him know how things were going. Terry made a tape for Tony using his own images, to be played prior to and during the surgery.

The Empowered Patient

As time for the surgery approached, Tony was very assertive about letting his doctor know what he needed. The surgical team was very supportive and very interested in this unusual partnership. The anesthesiologist added "changing the imagery/relaxation tapes" to his duties during the surgery!

A second tape was made as a result of another imagery session in which Tony rehearsed how he wanted the postoperative activities to progress. This tape was based on Terry's description of what activities to expect. Control of pain was also incorporated into the tape using Tony's images. The end of the tape focused on "seeing" the healing process. Tony saw "the little bone cells growing like coral, increasing in number and density" and imagined "the bone becoming stronger with each step as if there were a special signal with each step that encourages the healing process." Tony also future-paced this rehearsal to see himself six months away, walking without pain and without a limp.

Results

Tony stayed in the hospital for five days with minimal pain. His surgeon told him the operation took 20 percent less time than anticipated, probably due to Tony's relaxed state. Tony used the tapes from the imagery sessions as well as other relaxation tapes during surgery, throughout his hospitalization, and in the immediate postoperative period. He was able to squat in thirteen weeks and walk without a limp in four months. As of this writing, almost one year since surgery, Tony is well into an aggressive rehabilitation phase. He feels the imagery contributed significantly to his quick recovery.

Nurses can be instrumental in encouraging patients to participate and influence their surgical outcomes by using imagery and relaxation techniques.

Reminders

This is a beautiful example of what is possible in nursing. As healers, however, it is crucial that we value patients as special and honor their experiences equally. It is very important to give patients permission to use whatever they need medically.

Nurses can be instrumental in carrying through the patient's images from preoperative time through surgery and into recovery. It is very helpful for us to take the responsibility to pass on all valuable information to ensure consistency in care. This is another small example of the many ways in which nursing can make a big difference.

FINAL THOUGHTS: CREATING SACRED SPACE

We have already discussed the importance of helping the client to feel that he is in a safe place. The act of supporting this process is a healing gesture. A special place is sacred, giving the client a sense that he can escape from chronic pain and locate spiritual support.

When a client is having severe pain, the guide can suggest several methods and let the client select the one that feels most likely to help. In working with people in pain, the nurse will often notice that the pain shifts from one spot to another. It is important to stay with the client until he has achieved a sense of completion for the time being.

When we work with clients in this manner, we are imparting more than technique. We are offering them a potential to make healthy decisions. We are teaching them to think from the larger perspective. We are offering empowerment.

SUMMARY

There are many ways to become creative and inspired with these techniques. As you begin to incorporate them into your daily experiences, you will ascertain which ones are most enjoyable for you, and you will also gain expertise and be able to match clients and situations with the most effective tools.

Nurses using imagery in their work feel more creative and rejuvenated while they help to enhance the coping abilities and sense of control of their clients.

References

California Nurses Association. (1982, March). *Position statement: RN as provider of relaxation and suggestive therapies.* San Francisco: Author.

Dossey, L. (1993). *Healing words: The power of prayer and the practice of medicine.* New York: HarperCollins.

Newman, M. (1986). *Health as expanding consciousness.* St. Louis: C.V. Mosby.

6

CREATIVE IMAGERY: ADVANCED CLINICAL APPLICATIONS

Using imagery, the nurse can help the client make changes in perception and behavioral attitudes that can promote healing. . . . Nurses and clients come to know themselves in a new way as they create and communicate in a symbolic language.

Barbara M. Dossey, 1988

As we begin to consider more advanced possibilities for imagery in the clinical setting, we can be more creative. Once we understand the basic concepts and know how to help the client tap into his special place, we are able to move beyond technique and into creative applications.

There are several more advanced techniques. Beyond those techniques, there is a way of thinking that allows people undergoing major life transitions to feel more expansive and empowered. We will discuss some of the more sophisticated techniques first in this chapter. Later we will explore the ways in which the nurse can begin to tap into a creative exploration of the spiritual realm. Many of these advanced tools are extremely helpful for people who are facing crises, critical illnesses, or death.

WORKING WITH LIFE TRANSITIONS

When people are facing life-threatening illnesses, offering them a special place gives them a break from a very wearing and strained reality. Many of the techniques already mentioned can be quite helpful for their distraction effect, as well as for relaxation. There are ways to go deeper in this work with people facing birth and death. These ideas are explored to encourage nurses to create and touch their patients in the deepest, most meaningful way.

Remember that we are privileged to work with people making life transitions. This work is closely related to the ministry, and it is best approached with a reverent and sacred intent. The intent is the energy we devote to the situation and the attitude that we hold as we do our work. Working with imagery requires that we align our intent with the higher will, so that what needs to happen in any person's life will be supported.

PARTS WORK

Another helpful and rather advanced technique for working with images is to imagine the various parts of the self (physically or emotionally). This can be a very sophisticated process at times, and once again should be embarked upon by practitioners with additional training.

In parts work, the practitioner helps the client to acknowledge the many parts of himself. In doing this, there is a growing recognition that many of the parts are not aligned.

The practitioner might help the client to relax and deepen the relaxation, then progress to having the client see the various sides he is taking in facing a particular challenge. Each of these parts may have a voice and may say something that does not support or agree with other parts of the self. To become aware of inner conflict is to begin healing.

For example, consider the client who comes in for assistance with a long-standing chronic condition. In working with the client, it becomes apparent to the guide that the client feels he must remain ill in order to continue to collect disability payments from the state. The client might then be encouraged to see each of those parts arguing with the others, trying to reach some consensus about what to do. This work has also been referred to as *subpersonality work*. In the work, the client can imagine his different parts in different ways.

In one type of parts work, the client is encouraged to dialogue with the part of himself that is uncomfortable. If several parts are involved, he might imagine the parts in a variety of ways. He could picture the parts as a bunch of children on a school bus in which the bus driver is gone. One by one, the children take over driving the bus. Some are afraid and driving in the wrong direction because they fear the destination. Some are unafraid and drive in the opposite direction. Some, being aggressive, drive recklessly. Others are stubborn; they get behind the wheel, put on the brakes, and refuse to drive anywhere.

The client is encouraged to give each of these parts a chance to speak, be listened to, and be comforted, while keeping the good of the whole organism in mind. He can then be supported in allowing healing to transpire in each of the parts and in the entire scenario.

The client might see the part of himself that is afraid to get well, take responsibility for his life, and become independent. Working with and nurturing this part allows the client to cease judgment, integrate all of his parts, and feel more whole.

From this place of wholeness, better choices are made from a wider variety of options. It is particularly helpful to allow a client to stop judging his situation. We can often be our own worst critics. In healing work, the nurse can present a model of nonjudgmental caring, thus allowing the client to honor his process, and eventually to waste less time working against self-judgment and internal criticism.

As another example, a client may express ambivalent feelings about a procedure or decision. The practitioner can encourage him to get in touch with his parts, including the optimistic part, the fearful part, and the angry part.

Another revealing exercise might be to do an imagery experience, then draw the different parts of the self. This artistic expression of imagery experiences can be both revealing and cathartic.

Regression with Inner Guide

Some practitioners who are well-trained in this work can direct the parts to dialogue with each other. Others might choose to guide the client to a time when the fear was inspired. A therapist working with imagery might ask the client, "How old do you feel right now?," guiding the client to earlier times and working with the frightened inner child who needs comfort.

Regression with an inner guide is an advanced-level technique, something a nurse might look forward to if this type of work excites her. The addition of the inner guide to regression work adds something very beneficial—a safety net that can be pulled out in times of emotional emergency.

For example, a practitioner might be working with a client who has identified emotional problems. Certain topics may be extremely provocative, and the client might be directed to ask his inner guide whether to proceed and how. This safety net protects both the client and the practitioner from treading in dangerous areas. The inner guide can be the counselor who knows the client best and knows what he is capable of handling. In this way, the client never goes beyond his limits.

In regression with an inner guide, we might ask the inner guide, "What do you think we should look at?" If the inner guide says, "Go back to age five," the practitioner might ask, "Should we observe the child at age five or have him regress back to age five?"

Being five is a much deeper level than observing the five-year-old. Using the inner guide to determine which level to work with provides the safety net that could be the difference between trauma and insight.

Hypnosis has often been feared because it offers no such safety net. Hypnotists have often regressed people without their inner permission or agreement. In some of these instances, the person has encountered traumatic repressed material for which he was unprepared.

For some of these reasons, this type of work, delving into very deep levels, *must* be done by trained counselors. A nurse might refer the client to an imagery specialist, psychiatric clinical specialist, psychiatrist (in the hospital setting), or private counselor with excellent references.

Healing Another Part: The Inner Child Work

Recent years have seen an explosion in materials related to codependency issues. This has been mentioned in earlier parts of this book. Here we will explore imagery that might relate to powerful inner healing commonly referred to as working with the *inner child.*

Codependency experts have recently supported the growth of individuals beyond early life traumas by encouraging them to go back to the time when they were children experiencing emotional wounding. The client is asked to see that child (himself at an earlier time), communicate with the child, hold the child, and begin to offer the child protection. The client then gives his inner child whatever he missed in earlier life experiences.

This is a powerful inner way to heal the wounding. The client learns to be his own protector and advocate and is encouraged to return to visit his inner child frequently and regularly. By so doing, the client can bring the image forward in time to a place where the child is no longer emotionally stunted, but instead feels whole and loved.

This work can be extremely beneficial for people who have major areas in their lives where they seem to be stuck in childlike functioning. It is important to remember that there is a distinction between regression and visiting the younger self. The levels are very different and require the skills of an advanced imagery therapist. The return to the traumatic experience, coupled with the addition of self-nurturing and self-acceptance, can enhance a person's movement into a more mature level of functioning.

People do not often embark upon this level of work until they break through denial about aspects of their lives that are not working. Inner child work demands a willingness to face old hurts and to let them go and move beyond them. For these reasons, this type of work is often accomplished in conjunction with psychotherapy.

A therapist must have worked on and resolved many of her own childhood issues to be effective with this level of interaction. Inner child work is not intended for use by the novice who has not yet healed her own early trauma. Deep emotional catharsis can accompany these maneuvers, so they are best done when the setting allows for intense feelings to arise and be worked with therapeutically.

DANGER: PLANTING IMAGES CAN BE HAZARDOUS TO HEALTH

A note of caution is added here about judgment. As guides, we can support our clients' self-healing endeavors and attempt to inspire healthy attitudes. We can help them to get out of the way of their own inner healers.

It is not our job, however, to place any value judgment on our clients' lifestyles or decisions. We may wish to encourage their selection of healthy options, and we might point out ideas to expand their thought processes. We work with many cultures, many religions, and many belief systems. As was mentioned earlier, it is imperative that we remain open-minded to each client's process, and allow that client to grow in his timing, according to his beliefs.

Likewise, it is crucial that we encourage the client to supply the images as much as possible. If we come across as heavy-handed, critical, or frightening in any way, we will not only lose the trust of the client, but will also dampen his enthusiasm for his own healing process.

Healing is a very individualized endeavor. What works for one client may not be at all appropriate for another. We need to take time to know our clients and to allow them to supply the ideas as much as possible for their journeys to wholeness.

Of particular concern at this time is the raging controversy about the therapist's ability to influence the client negatively. Recent newspaper and journal articles debate the "false memory syndrome," which allows for a sudden return of emotional experience that has been buried for many years in the subconscious mind.

In many such instances, a person literally wakes up one day with a vivid recollection of something horrible, something that has affected him mentally, emotionally, and physically for much of his lifetime. It may be a memory that has been buried in the subconscious mind for years.

There are some memory experts who have studied this phenomenon and are helpful in deciding in which cases the memory is accurate (all physical evidence may have disappeared years ago). The expert may have to rely on circumstantial evidence, noting how the behavior of the person is consistent or inconsistent with someone who has undergone that particular trauma.

This type of work is extremely delicate, because many of the memories are of life and death incidents that could necessitate legal intervention.

In the midst of these raging battles, a practitioner must exhibit extreme caution and sensitivity to deep emotional issues that may arise. Some patients have reported having memories that may have been suggested by an ambitious or influential counselor, and this phenomenon has resulted in major upheaval in the courts.

The therapist may have her own ideas about what might have happened to a client, but these ideas do not belong to the client, they belong to the therapist. They should remain with the therapist for the client's sake and for the purity of the process.

RE-EVALUATION OF PAST TRAUMA (REFRAMING)

In having a neutral person with whom to share ideas, the client may also gain an opportunity to take another look at a past experience from a new vantage point. When a client is deeply relaxed, travels mentally to a safe place, and enlists the assistance of his inner guide, he may be led to new ideas and images to replace some of the previously distressing ones.

For example, a client may have been working for years in counseling with the traumatic sudden death of a parent when he was young. He may have worked with his deep grief, his rage, and his sense of abandonment. At some point, however, he may come to see the power of the gift he was given.

Many powerful healers had similar traumatic experiences in their youth and have been able to use their inner guidance to view the opportunities they were granted once they completed a major part of the grieving work. Again, the inner guide can be used for safety to ascertain how to progress.

Similarly, as practitioners, we might choose to redirect a client's attention to the positive results gained through this major life event. This is not to say we should in any way stifle any grieving or anger that arises, but rather that at some point, we should help the person become better equipped to accept the experience and grow from it. We can support this process by allowing the space for this reframing to occur.

AGE PROGRESSIONS (REHEARSAL)

Similar to age regressions, we can enlist the deeply relaxed state to bring a client forward in time. This technique is often administered as a form of positive rehearsal. For example, we might use this on a convalescing postmastectomy patient, asking her to look at what she wants. She might specify that she wishes to see herself doing very well in the future. The practitioner may use guided imagery or allow the patient's images to surface.

In a guided session, the practitioner may progress in the following manner: "Now you are five years postmastectomy. You have done very, very well. You look back on five years of complete comfort, with no cancer recurrence. You are enjoying wonderful health; you're feeling good about how it all transpired. You recognize how strong your immune system is, and you appreciate its magnificent contributions to your sense of wholeness and well-being. You see all the people who have supported you on this journey. You feel their love and send your love back to them. You deeply appreciate yourself as a major player in your healing work, and give thanks to your Higher Power, however you see that power."

In this way, the nurse can guide the patient to think positively and help her to handle the fears that will naturally arise. The patient is also building immunity by seeing herself as strong and healthy.

This kind of visual imagery has been used in many treatment programs, as well as in athletic and business endeavors. It is positive rehearsal that inspires a happy, healthy body-mind environment.

SPIRITUAL NURSING CARE

Many of the ideas mentioned in this chapter cross the line from specific application of skills to spiritual counseling. These are most useful to nurses who feel comfortable with a holistic approach and are accustomed to incorporating the spiritual dimension of healing into their work. All tools are not for everyone.

For nurses who do not yet feel competent to work in this way, there are many ways to begin to prepare for this high-level work. Consider becoming involved with holistic nursing organizations and read books that support this model (see Appendix). A certificate program in Holistic Nursing is offered through the American Holistic Nurses Association.

General Spiritual Growth

As the person begins to think more positively, there is an alignment of the human being with the inner person, the soul, or source. In this view, there is an assumption that people are more than their bodies; we are multidimensional beings who operate on many levels at once. The holistic practitioner works with people to support the alignment and integration of their various levels.

In this viewpoint, as discussed in the previous section, a client might choose to see his illness or disease as a "kick in the pants," an incentive to start making some healthy changes. In this process, the client may utilize any information received through relaxation processes to help get back on his growth tract.

If a client chooses to view an experience as soul expanding, he may use it to realign himself with the spiritual purpose, his life path. In this manner, he may view himself as evolving in consciousness, for he may incorporate the old information in new ways through expanding thought processes.

Whatever the client chooses to believe about his place in the higher order of life, he can use this opportunity to feel closer to the source of his life and his soul's desire. Growth in the spiritual realm allows people to live and die more peacefully.

As we face the AIDS epidemic, we witness more bright, young, articulate people facing death. These people are teaching us that healing is a multilayered experience, of which death is a natural part. We can help them and ourselves to face all of life's passages with dignity and trust.

The Healing Circle

Another powerful technique, more intermediate than advanced, but included here under spiritual aspects, is known as the Healing Circle. The nurse guides the patient to his special place and has him imagine that he is surrounded by all of his favorite animals or objects. This type of emotive imagery elicits a deep sense of love and support in the patient. All people want to feel loved, and this is true even more so when they are facing illness or death.

You might encounter people who have never experienced a great deal of support. These clients, without the benefit of memory to carry them through, must be enticed to use their creative imagination. Even if they have never experienced something, clients can use mind power to imagine it!

Have the client picture loved ones as everything he ever dreamed could exist, or however he yearned for them to be. Guide the client to share his most intimate feelings with someone he wished could have loved him as much as he loved that person. Have him breathe in the love he envisions, have him feel it and let it warm his heart and soul. Support him in feeling fulfilled and nourished.

Past Life Regressions

Many hypnotists have been surprised in working with patients to discover that the patients have lapsed into some other realm. These patients may start talking about events that seem out of time, and are somehow from another era or another place. Many people believe that these spontaneous events are a result of time traveling to another lifetime. Others, however, believe that the patient has tapped into what Jung called the *collective unconscious.*

When working with people who believe in past life regression, the most profound healing often occurs by helping the client to find a framework for his life that puts all events into a meaningful system. It is preferable that a guide offer this type of assistance, rather than have the client try to make literal sense of the symbols and images that arise.

Just as in working with dreams, the symbology in past life regression can be very personal. Healing transpires when the client can use the material in some meaningful way. It is best that the evolving guide allow the meaning to arise from the client's wellspring of feelings and life events, rather than try to interpret.

Higher Sense Perception

Highly creative individuals can expand their awareness to contact others by tapping into what Jung called the "collective consciousness." There are many other ways to expand awareness and interconnection, including developing the art of clairvoyance (highly developed sight, allowing for the ability to see subtle energies), clairaudience (hearing beyond the usual ability, including the ability to hear subtle energy sounds), and what is commonly known as astral traveling (transporting the soul from one location to another).

All of these abilities rely on the dedicated development of what is called *higher sense perception*. In focusing on subtle energies, people can become adept at noticing sensations that normally escape the common attention.

Parapsychology and physics have expanded the realm of what is considered possible in recent years, pushing the edges of acceptability farther into previously uncharted territory.

Energetic research has provided evidence of the existence of subtle energy flows and the ability to influence physiological responses through touch and energy field interactions. Energy centers (chakras), which exchange energy between the layers of the energy field and interface with the physical body, have been identified.

Awareness of these structures and their effects on vitality and well-being can enhance the imagery healing endeavors. For example, if a client has identified patterns of disease related to specific body areas, he might imagine the chakra for that area. He can ask for an image of the chakra and work with the image that arises. He might also envision how it needs to look to be healthy and invite that image to represent his center.

The book *Healing Touch* provides thorough descriptions of energy field phenomenon (Hover-Kramer, 1995).

Contacting Physical and Nonphysical Guidance

It has long been considered that extrasensory perception (ESP) exists, accounting for the ability of people to sense the energies of others whether near or far apart. As a guide in healing endeavors, the nurse might also find herself in the position of trying to help the patient contact significant others, near or far.

Nurses are often at the bedside in times of major life transitions, and we can provide enormous support by assisting the patient in tapping into whatever resources he can identify to adequately survive life challenges.

Healing a Previous Loss Through Imagery

One nurse told of caring for a woman who was having a difficult labor. In working with the woman's images, it became apparent that her labor was intensified due to the emotionality of having birthed a child years ago that she had given up for adoption. As she proceeded with labor, she felt increasingly guilty and pained, recalling the last time she had given birth and how painful those buried memories were as they surfaced.

The nurse encouraged the woman to envision her adopted child and to know that all was fine for that child. The nurse spoke in soothing tones, inviting the laboring woman to make contact with the first child and ask for forgiveness. The woman received an image of a happy, healthy girl who was playing in the woods and was very in touch with nature. The woman asked her adopted daughter to forgive her, something she had never been able to face before, and broke into a large smile as the image of the girl laughed and giggled and hugged her.

The woman was able to feel as if she were truly in contact with the soul of her first child for the first time, and she felt a deep sense of inner peace and completion. Knowing in her heart that she had done the best she could, and that she had done the right thing, the woman was able to release the emotionality of the past and free herself to fully experience the birth of her second child.

As nurses, there are countless ways to be creative in using the imagination to support the healing work of our clients. Inspiration for the healing work will often arise from the client himself, particularly if the nurse can be gentle in her approach and listen carefully to the unspoken or whispered visions of the client.

Too often we allow the noise and commotion of the modern hospital environment to dictate the pace and quality of attention we give. In using imagery in creative ways, we give ourselves and our clients a highly valued gift—the chance to reconnect with the true inner self.

When we learn to listen and to carefully honor the inner voices within ourselves and our patients, we open ourselves to a whole new dimension in patient care. The small, still voice that speaks in the silence brings powerful information that could come in no other way. The wisdom of the soul enlightens our work, lighting the path for new directions and expanded meaning in all that we do. We can learn, as healers, to take our directions from the subtle influences arising from quiet moments in relaxed states.

Creating Healing Teams

There are many ways to enlist the support of helpers as we blaze new trails on the road to recovery. There are likely to be as many ways to heal as there are people in the world.

Some individuals believe in consulting the most renowned experts on their journey. For these people, they might call in the best surgeons, medicine men or women, or other specialists to provide their care. Others may research thoroughly, reading everything they can find on certain topics. They might use computers to locate all related articles, purchase every book written about their diseases, and perhaps even find papers at the National Archives or National Institutes of Health Library.

Still others might make a point of locating any people who were in their positions and beat the odds. They might read about these exceptional patients or make contact with them by joining groups or contacting individuals.

A further extension of this approach was offered by the nurse who told us that she had a patient challenging AIDS who spent many hours in quiet contemplation. No one was aware of what he was doing until she took the risk of asking the patient what he did in all his quiet time. The patient was delighted to share his process, and the nurse learned a magnificent tool from him.

John

John had studied the writings of the well-known author Napoleon Hill. In one of his books, Napoleon Hill (1987) mentioned that he had created his own "mental cabinet," a committee dedicated to helping him through modeling wisdom, courage, and other traits that he desired for himself. He held imaginary meetings regularly with his cabinet members and solicited their advice for daily decisions. These meetings, according to Mr. Hill, became so real that he was able to make excellent decisions on many aspects of his existence.

John was very impressed with this approach. When he received his diagnosis of AIDS, he decided that he would work creatively with his own "cabinet," seeking support and wisdom from a self-selected group of healers. Some of the advisors in his cabinet were great healers from all times; and others were people he had known or still knew. Some were alive, some were dead, some were imaginary.

John's healing team could expand or contract to meet the needs of every moment, and he found great solace in surrounding himself mentally with loving presences, all of whom had much to offer to him as he faced his lonely healing journey.

In working with John, the nurse witnessed his incredible faith. She was deeply touched and inspired by his spirit and the integrity with which he approached his mission. It was obvious to all who came into contact with John that his was not a situation of dying, but instead was a growth into life.

John inspired all who knew him, not because of the outcome of his illness, but because of his approach to it. He credited his tremendous courage to the fact that he was so supported by his healing team. And to think his healing team was all his creation, in his mind, in his way. This is what made it so empowering; John had designed his healing process. It was easy and enjoyable for the nurses to work with John because he felt surrounded by love and strength.

Avoiding Negative Influence

Conversely, there have been healing programs designed for people challenging chronic or life-threatening illnesses which specifically deny the patients' access to the media. These experiments have been very interesting in that they encourage people to monitor the input, or media communication, while being taxed by severe illnesses. Input can be immune building or immune depleting.

Radio, television news, and newspapers, with their overly negative images and reports, have been considered to contribute to the immune depletion many people experience. It stands to reason that negative images are perceived as stressful when we consider that positive images enhance immune responses.

For this reason, people involved in healing work might consider the impact of all images and experiences, both immune

enhancing and depleting, prior to exposure. It can be good medicine to weigh carefully the benefits of any activities versus the
potential detriment to one's health and well-being.

When we as health providers make conscious decisions
about our health, we are also serving as models to our clients.
For these reasons, it is immeasurably helpful for nurses to
change their perceptions of their work.

The media has not been particularly sensitive to nursing's
issues and has often portrayed the nurse negatively. Nurses are
now challenged to change their mental imagery about their work
to inspire further changes in the health care delivery system in
which we have been operating.

Imagery in the Face of Death

Imagery can be used in infinitely creative ways. We have mentioned the guided visual approach to challenging cancer, the work
by the Simontons. There are people who are taking imagery far
beyond the Simonton approach. Many people challenging AIDS
consider that they are harnessing their immune birthright and
imagine themselves whole and perfect.

For others, the question arises as to when to continue the
fight and when to gracefully come to grips with mortality. There
has been an explosion of books in recent years that deal with
honoring the dying process.

Particularly for those challenging the AIDS epidemic, people
have embarked upon intense soul searching to find answers that
are not readily accessible. Some practitioners working with the
large gay community in the San Francisco area have encouraged
the people challenging AIDS to answer some difficult questions.
"What programming about being gay might have dampered your
immune enthusiasm?" "What alienation/degradation has tarnished
your ability to mount a proper offense?"

In struggling to find answers to life's more dire challenges,
people must be willing to look honestly into their own psyches,
and to tell the truth. For most people, this is a terrifying and
difficult process. We have been acculturated to deny the painful
aspects of lives, often choosing to turn our backs on the realities
and conjure up reasons that protect us from our deepest feelings.

People facing life-threatening illnesses do not have the luxury of denial. Time is often limited, and there is much to accomplish for healing to occur. Working with people in this position is an honor, because it forces us to face our deeper fears as well. In these instances, our patients become our teachers, and we learn to be honest in our lives.

Autoimmune Imagery

There are also a variety of ways in which people challenging autoimmune disorders can image their illness. We will consider a creative and helpful approach by Dr. Richard Shames, a general practitioner in Mill Valley, CA, who works with many people challenged by thyroid disorders. In working with autoimmune thyroiditis (Hashimoto's disease), Shames has learned to identify the health situations of his patients graphically.

In Hashimoto's disease, the immune system identifies the thyroid gland as a foreign body, causing the immune cells to attack the gland. The result is inflammation and a multitude of related symptoms. Dr. Shames suggests that his patients consider "calling the dogs off the mailman." He advises his patients that the immune system has become so zealous in its protection function that it starts eating away organs.

What image might help? Dr. Shames suggests that the patient round up the pack of dogs that protect his home from unwanted intruders and have a good hard talk with them about leaving the mailman alone. Shames suggests that the patient make sure the dogs understand that he is *not* an intruder; in fact, the dogs should know that the patient needs them.

There are many other autoimmune diseases that operate similarly. In rheumatoid arthritis, the immune system attacks cartilage. In diabetes, the islet cells of the pancreas are attacked.

A milder version of this same response is allergy. The overzealous immune system must be encouraged to tone down, turn the volume down a notch or two, and realize that the world is a great place.

It can be helpful to remember that the Creator put all things on earth for us to revel in. Pollen and dust are part of the cycle of nature that we are a part of, and we can choose to see them as nonthreatening.

Even molds and mites are a part of the great mystery of life. We can learn to comfortably coexist with all life forms and to love ourselves. We all share the planet. We can learn to share with greater grace and equanimity.

Beyond Fear

This new way of thinking takes us to another level of functioning in our lives. We can begin to approach the world as Dr. Gerald Jampolsky (1979) has recommended, filled with love rather than filled with fear.

This level of information assures us that there are ultimate fears that must be faced head-on. These include the fear of being alone, the fear of dying without having lived fully, the fear of never being loved as one wishes to be loved. Nonetheless, we can learn to meet these fears with a sense of peacefulness.

Anger and Health

We are further encouraged to consider the role of anger in our lives. Anger is not healthy if we hold on to it. It is an emotion to be felt and expressed in a safe, productive manner. Most people have not learned to honor and discharge anger healthily.

Consider the person challenging high blood pressure. To heal thoroughly, he may need to consider the source of his anger. He might also have an opportunity to make some different decisions about how he chooses to live.

One advanced technique for overcoming the ill effects of anger is to let it be okay that people are the way they are. Years ago in co-counseling classes, the motto was "The world's the way it is, and people are the way they are—and that's the way it is!"

Here is an exercise for people who have difficulty expressing anger. These people often generate high blood pressure. In working with someone who fits this category, consider the following guided imagery:

Tell the patient that in his imagination, he can go up to the person he is angry with and let him have it; he can blast him with anger and be as animated, evocative, forceful, dramatic, and furious as he wants to be. Then he can see that person giving an appropriate response, perhaps a long-overdue apology. Have the client then see himself feeling relieved and experiencing reconciliation and a deep level of healing.

This process can offer tremendous relief to people caught in certain emotional dramas. It can also be used for someone with unfinished business with a deceased person. There is often a sense of expansion in doing this exercise, which allows the person to move forward in his life at long last.

Playing Detective

Here is another "game" that encourages people to look at their situations differently, perhaps even to enjoy the prospect of reclaiming health. Have the client imagine that there is one clue that is the key to the whole case, something that has been overlooked by the doctors and therapists involved. As a good detective, with the help of the inner advisor (who might be seen with a Sherlock Holmes hat and looking glass), run through every aspect of this malady with the idea that you will uncover the clue that will bust the case wide open and turn it around. Imagine how much fun it can be to take charge of your health and be your own healer!

Spiritual Uses of Imagery

These are some examples of advanced techniques. The more advanced one becomes, the more one delves into the spiritual realm. Krishnamurti, a spiritual teacher, was understood to have said that beginning practice is rather rote; one follows it precisely. As one grows in wisdom, understanding, and experience, one develops one's own style.

As a nurse incorporating imagery, these ideas might be slightly different than you were taught. You might begin to individualize that style for the clients you work with. You may even develop your own advanced techniques, ones that make sense to you and your clients in your particular time and setting.

This is advanced imagery. This is what differentiates between a technician performing simple exercises and a high-level, knowledgeable healer. The basic interventions often relate strictly to the body level, the intermediate interventions might also address mental or emotional levels. The advanced practice tends to work with matters of the spirit as well as physical and mental/emotional levels. The holistic imagery practitioner works on a multidimensional basis, allowing her creativity to blend with that of the client, inspiring new levels of understanding, acceptance, and wellness.

Keep in mind that the beginning practitioner does not use these techniques without further training, though they are presented to entice the practitioner. Also remember that some techniques will appeal to you more than others.

A wide range of ideas has been introduced in this section largely to demonstrate the enormous flexibility of this tool and the potential for creative nursing endeavors.

HEALING OF THE ETHERIC BODY

As we have seen, advanced healings do not have to deal simply with the physical body or psychological dynamics. There are more subtle bodies surrounding the physical, and these can be enhanced by imagery to provide very powerful healing.

For example, in the Healing Touch Certification program offered through the American Holistic Nurses Association (see Appendix), nurses learn to sense the various layers of the human energy field. They can then bring the client into alignment by having him visualize his chakras, or energy centers.

The nurse can be instrumental in sharing this high-level information with clients who are prepared to receive it. Not all nurses will want to work on these subtle levels with clients. Also, not all clients will want to assume this level of responsibility for their evolving wellness. For those who are eager to participate in their healing, however, these tools are invaluable and empowering.

Once the nurse has taught the client about the various energy centers, the nurse can encourage the client to imagine his own chakras, paying attention to which ones are open, closed, spinning, or leaking energy. The self-actualized client can further be taught to repair his energy field. He can also be reminded to call upon his healing team, complete with all helpers.

Working on these levels borders on the mystical and spiritual levels, and once again is not intended for all clients or all practitioners. The information is presented for those who wish to move beyond ordinary medical care and to experiment with human energy interactions.

ONENESS WITH THE UNIVERSE

Spiritual alignment allows one to feel more unified in his entirety (body-mind-spirit). Aligning with universal energy allows access to the healing power of the universe. Clients can be guided to view themselves as part of the healing universe, rather than separate from it.

For example, the client might be told: "Your atoms are the atoms of the mountains and oceans. Keep in mind that you, the mountains, and the oceans are the dust of previously exploded stars that have congealed on this planet. When we think about it, we are all stardust, part of the universal flow of matter, part of the enormous giant divine plan.

"Allow yourself to experience the comfort of the larger view of all these phenomenon. When we take the time to consider the largest picture, it becomes more clear that the universe is unfolding exactly as it should. Each of us remembers that we are held in the bosom of the Great Mother. We can feel our pulse in line with the pulse of the galaxy, and know that we are living in the flow of life, and that we are holy, and connected, and loved.

"These thoughts can bring us through many of life's darker moments. We choose where our mind focuses; let us consider channeling the power of the mind to create beauty and harmony for all life forms."

SUMMARY

Techniques and approaches to advanced-level imagery can be infinitely creative and resourceful. The nurse who is inspired may rejuvenate herself through enhanced creativity while she works uniquely with each patient using imagery.

References

Dossey, B., Keegan, L., Guzzetta, C., & Kolkmeier, L. (1988). *Holistic nursing: A handbook for practice.* Rockville, MD: Aspen Publishers, Inc.

Dossey, L. (1994). *Healing words: The power of prayer and the practice of medicine.* San Francisco: HarperCollins.

Hill, N. (1987). *Think and grow rich.* New York: Fawcett.

Hover-Kramer, D. (1995). *Healing touch: A resource for health care professionals.* New York: Delmar Publishers.

Jampolsky, G. (1979). *Love is letting go of fear.* Millbrae, CA: Celestial Arts.

Newman, M. (1986). *Health as expanding consciousness.* St. Louis: C.V. Mosby Company.

INTEGRATION INTO NURSING PRACTICE

7

INTERVIEWS: NURSES WITH IMAGINATION

You can accomplish anything if you do not accept limitations . . . Whatever you make up your mind to do, you can do.

Paramahansa Yogananda, 1946

We have explored imagery definitions and history. We have described techniques nurses can use to incorporate imagery into their practices. We have examined situations that can benefit from introducing relaxation and visualization. We have also considered how the nurse can begin to use imagery for her own self-healing.

To consolidate much of this material, to have it come alive and be more meaningful, the author interviewed several nurses who have expanded their practices through the use of imagery and visualization. Some of the nurses, in addition to using imagery in their nursing practices, have used imagery to heal themselves. The following is a distillation of their wisdom and interviews.

INTRODUCTORY IDEAS OF NURSE/IMAGERY SPECIALISTS

An Interview with Three Nurses

(The following material is excerpted from an interview in the spring of 1994 with Karilee Halo Shames, RN, PhD; Susan Ezra, RN; and Jan Maxwell, RN, BA in Dr. Shames' Mill Valley office.)

"The imagery process can be very simple. We always tell our patients that if they can worry, they are already practicing imagery. (Worry is a process of imagining a negative outcome in a future event and responding mentally and physiologically to the negative images before the actual event ever occurs.)

"As nurses, we are so very busy that it is easy to get lost in tasks; we can be readily overwhelmed. In this mental state, it would be likely that we would look upon the prospect of providing imagery as one more burdensome task. It is important to realize that we can begin to incorporate segments of this work in minute doses. The intent is to ease pressure, not to create more.

"As an example, if you are working postoperatively and administering antibiotics into the IV of a lucid, cooperative patient, you might suggest that he imagine the medication entering the bloodstream, flowing through the capillaries and vessels, delivering a perfect dose to eliminate bacteria. It is useful to keep the suggestions small and simple.

"Remember that people are very suggestible when they are feeling vulnerable, and our words are influential. For this reason, classical hypnosis has often incorporated preoperative hypnotic suggestions to influence the course of surgery.

"For any procedure, the nurse can suggest that the patient 'think of a vacation place.' This is very simple yet transformative when people are under duress.

"Often people are not breathing enough; when we are in a state of fear and contracted, we often stop our full, deep breathing that could allow for a release and relaxation. The nurse can remind the client to breathe, encouraging him to take slow, deep breaths. At times, it is helpful to be even more specific, especially if the client seems highly anxious.

"The nurse can breathe deeply with the client, emphasizing the inspirations and expirations, which also allows for some nurse relaxation! She might also, with the client's understanding and permission, gently place her hand on the client's abdomen and have him breathe into that area. As nurses, we have license to touch, and it is quite natural to combine touch with soothing words.

"It is also critical that the nurse remember that imagery is not only referring to that which is seen; rather, imagery is considered to be thought with sensory qualities. All senses, including sight, sound, smell, touch, and taste, can be involved in imagery process.

The Nurse's Role

"Keep in mind that the essence of nursing is to facilitate the healing process, even as described in various writings by Florence Nightingale in the mid-1800s. She spoke to the need for us to learn to facilitate the process of others, rather than to do things for them.

"We must recall that our clients are each endowed with infinite resources within. We are like the gardeners, watering the soil and nurturing the tender plant so it can grow. We do not make it grow; we help it to grow. It is difficult for nurses to get out of the helping mentality, but when we do that, we empower our clients and our work."

Concerns About Emotional Safety

"There are many ways to help clients access information, yet part of our skill involves developing the ability to match the techniques to the people. Some of the very powerful processes available for healing would not be helpful with certain populations. We must always use our nursing judgment and pay attention to the clues our clients give us."

Jan Maxwell tells the story of a client who was prescribed Elavil for five years because he was depressed. In talking with him only a short while, it seemed evident that a major part of his depression was related to his not having grieved his wife's death. He had many physical symptoms, felt a great deal of pain, and needed opportunities to release emotionally. For this reason, relaxation imagery might not have been effective for this man until he had an opportunity to do grief work.

Special Considerations

Many issues that are highly charged emotionally arise with our patients. The nurse wishing to incorporate imagery into her practice must be aware of the potential concerns a patient might have and be willing to address them.

When working with a client using imagery, it is valuable to consider that the client may fear uncovering scary images. Most of us have the ability to develop very sophisticated defense mechanisms to avoid feeling enormous pain or despondency. A psychiatric nurse might be well-trained in supporting the release of intense emotional energy, but most nurses are not taught to handle these situations. Each nurse must respect her levels of competency and comfort.

The nurse is well-advised to always let her clients know that this work is self-guided. Tell the client that he is always in control and that he can freely choose to change the image or distance himself by opening his eyes and moving around.

Exercise

It is always safe to start with a relaxation. The nurse can then encourage the patient to dialogue with his symptoms on a conscious level. This can be very powerful and humorous at times, and it is often quite revealing. As an example, the nurse might say, "Mr. Smith, if your stomach could talk, what would it say?"

This simple technique can offer profound insight; it is as if one part of the client is having a conversation with another part of himself. The answers reveal some deeply held knowledge that has not come to the awareness in any other way.

Similarly, the nurse can suggest that the client draw his headache (after supplying him with materials). A frequently used technique is to have the client draw with his non-dominant hand, which allows the other side of the brain to be activated.

The nurse can proceed a step by suggesting that the client then draw his headache as he would like it to be. These simple, playful tools can help people discover new healing directions for themselves.

Body-Mind Nursing

In her attempts to support the integration of body-mind-spirit in her patients, the nurse often finds herself developing her creativity. As mentioned earlier, to facilitate the healing process, the nurse is encouraged to use foresight, insight, and hindsight.

With *foresight*, the nurse prepares well. She sets the scene comfortably, gets permission from the client, and pays attention to any signs of anxiety or distress.

With *insight*, the nurse introduces the process and provides an induction and the opportunity for relaxation. The safe atmosphere, coupled with the guidance, allows the client to gain insight into the situation.

With *hindsight*, the nurse goes through a debriefing with the client. She might ask him, "What did you learn?" and "How do you feel?" She might also look upon her experiences to ascertain how to proceed for future endeavors.

Utilizing Client Resources

It is important to gather all resources as we support people on critical journeys with life and death issues. The role of the mind is crucial in the healing process. For that reason, it is best to know about your patient's beliefs and to try to incorporate meaningful experiences into his care.

Another example of creativity in nursing is provided by Jan Maxwell. Jan had a client who spoke frequently of the angels who he felt continually guided him. In working with this gentleman, Jan invited the client's guides to help direct the client to his healing. It is always worthwhile to tap into the client's belief system and allow his beliefs to support the work.

Imagery can help connect the person to spiritual resources. It can serve to reconnect a person with a sense of self relative to the universe. This type of healing happens with open, accepting care, as has traditionally been reserved for clergy. However, remember that nursing's roots are highly intertwined with religion, and that part of our work is to nourish and feed the soul.

Special Thoughts from Susan Ezra

"Beyond Ordinary Nursing" (the imagery workshop for nurses mentioned previously) is our attempt to show nurses how to use imagery to facilitate healing. As we learn to use these tools to work on our own healing, we gain better positions to guide others through their healing processes. It is a co-process; we are on our own healing journey.

"Imagery does not have to be a difficult, complicated technique. It is a way the mind works in its ability to enhance the process. It is not an outside thing; it is an innate process to be utilized.

"If we know how to worry, we're already using the process. We can take it to a higher level. It's so easy to get caught up in tasks and lists. Most nurses think that to add anything new would be overwhelming. Little segments can be incorporated in doing blood pressures or IVs.

"For example, a person receiving IV antibiotics can imagine the medication moving through the bloodstream and traveling to where it's needed. People are vulnerable in these situations; it's important that we give them simple, positive images.

"A lot of my hospice patients want simple images to work with. They don't have a lot of energy for anything complicated. I always start with a relaxation technique. I never do inner advisor work, or dialogue with a symptom, or go back to a past event that has potential for escalating until I have done a relaxation and have had a chance to experience the patient's level of comfort or anxiety.

"When someone comes in for surgery, we can easily give him positive suggestions that he can use to influence the process. Nurses and anesthetists can do this easily.

"We need to remember that imagery may not be the best way to work with all patients all the time. There are many accesses to what I call the *core*. We can get to the core through touch therapies, psychotherapy, or various therapy combinations. Some people are more receptive than others to using these modalities.

"These techniques must be used with caution when working with patients who have difficulty distinguishing images from reality. When people are on antipsychotic drugs, they sometimes become very uncomfortable if they suddenly access their emotions after years of repressing. It is best for these clients to work with psychiatrically trained practitioners.

"Some people cannot allow themselves a deep state of relaxation without experiencing emotional release. For people in this condition, we can use artwork or some form of centering and movement therapy as a way to indirectly access emotions.

"In our training from the Academy, as we mentioned earlier, we work with the model of foresight, insight, and hindsight. Part of the foresight is to ask if the person would like to be involved in this process. This is part of our nursing observation. Insight is the process itself, relaxation then imagery process. Hindsight is the debriefing. 'How was it?' 'How do you feel?' This is a very complete model.

"We have documentation that these tools help. Studies have shown that using imagery reduces the necessity for high dosages of medication. This kind of continued study is crucial to impart the special contributions of the gentle healing modalities.

"The foundations of psychoneuroimmunology (PNI) are critical to this work as well: how the nervous system and immune system are influenced by thoughts and images and how the mind and body do relate to each other. This is the framework from which all applications are built.

"This is actually very ancient wisdom. In going back to this knowledge base, we are changing our perspective. We may have technological advantages, but the philosophy, feeling, and intent are quite similar. It took PNI to make it believable to the minds of Western practitioners. Our technology enabled us to prove the value of these ancient tools.

"I feel that nurses need to understand and appreciate the holistic model of care to effectively use this tool. I know some nurses who are ingrained in the physical care to the exclusion of any other areas. It seems valuable to have nurses know the gifts of holistic thinking, where we consider the total person by working with him on the level of body-mind-spirit synergy.

"One of my patients is a physician who has cancer. After all the other therapies, he told me that he believes that the magic is what will help him heal, not the medicine. His illness has taught him the more meaningful levels of existence.

"I have been working outside hospitals for thirteen years. I use these tools with hospice patients. I do get quite a few referrals from the staff at hospice to do imagery with patients and families from hospice.

"I find that my private imagery practice energizes me quite a bit more than my regular hospice work. I would not, however, want to work full time doing this level of visualization work. I can only do so much. I have noticed that after a certain amount of intimate process, I have a tendency to pick up my patient's pain. That would be overwhelming. Part of doing this work is knowing one's limits.

"There is great challenge in being in private practice. As an RN, I am not able to bill insurance for reimbursement. I ask clients to pay per session or to get an order from their physician for RN sessions for stress management, relaxation session, or coping with illness (if they want to try to get insurance reimbursement). I give them a statement for the session. Some of the insurance companies will pay for part of this treatment. We really need to push for nurse reimbursement for healing modalities.

"I am proud to practice holistically. I have finally learned to acknowledge that I do know a great deal about what I'm doing. I know I'm making a difference, and that feels wonderful. We can each make our contributions in our own way."

Special Thoughts from Jan Maxwell

"I once knew a nurse who assisted at IV pyelograms. When people were nervous, she would simply encourage them to imagine that they were in a place they really liked. That was it. And just that small bit of imagery really helped those people to experience the procedure more comfortably.

"Another simple technique she used was to tell the person to put his hand over the most affected area, or she put her hand there also, and then she encouraged the person to breathe into that space.

"Keep in mind that imagery is sensory; touch is part of that process. All the senses come into play in imagery. Most nursing practice allows for touch; it's natural to combine visualization and touch. The more senses we can invite to participate, the greater the potential for healing.

"As we mentioned earlier, I have found that I learn a lot by asking the simple question, 'If your stomach (or whatever is affected) could talk, what might it say?' This tells me a lot about the person.

"I can also give the person some drawing supplies, and ask him to draw the image. I might then ask him to draw what he would like the image to look like. In these simple ways, we discover much about the person, and more importantly, we allow him to discover for himself the power of his creative mind. This is how we support his empowerment. We like to support the concept of body-mind nursing, conveying the idea that there is no separation between these parts of ourselves.

"I think it's sometimes a challenge for nurses to get out of the rescuing healing mode. We have been so codependent that we seem to prefer helping others rather than trying to heal ourselves. Nurses wishing to use these tools often find that they must initially learn to be more centered, less involved in the patient's process, and more involved in taking better care of themselves.

"I remember when my sister-in-law had to go in for repeat foot surgery. It was the kind of operation where they would make decisions after they got in there and could see what was happening. She believes that she has guides, unseen helpers, who support her in her life. At that time, she asked her guides to watch over the process, to help the doctors and enable them to make the best decisions. In this way, she felt more in charge and less afraid.

"Most people are in a prayer mode when undergoing these major experiences. This is a perfect time to help them access their creativity and intuition. I can envision a time when the imagery nurse is part of the healing team in hospitals, helping people to undergo life transitions with their special skills.

"I think the idea of spirituality is that it reconnects a person with himself, and to the universe around him. It is a process of opening. There is a certain degree of fear, or timidity, when nurses consider dealing with the realm of the sacred. We think that anything having to do with this work belongs to the clergy, yet as holistic nurses, we are very much involved with the spirit.

"There are particular imagery approaches that seem especially suited to nurses. I recall that when I learned the technique of dialoguing with the symptoms, I knew that this was a special technique for nurses.

"Some people say that I must not be a nurse, because I work outside of hospitals. I tell them that I'm more of a nurse than I've ever been.

"I work under the umbrella of stress management counseling, but I also consider that I do holistic counseling. I'm blessed with a rich diversity, so there is an interesting variety and nice balance. I have an officemate, and we take turns using the space, so that is built-in insurance that I won't overwork. My client load runs from six to twelve people weekly.

"I have some very long-term clients that come back year after year to work on different life and health issues. Others come in for brief transitional help.

"As for beginning to incorporate imagery into nursing practice, I encourage nurses to try a piece at a time. Try it, practice with it, then try adding something new when you feel comfortable. Confidence comes first with finding the courage to take the risk, then trying something else and learning from every opportunity. In this way, we become leaders and serve as role models.

"It's different than telling a patient about doctor's orders. It might be scarier, because it's new and different. We need to experiment and see what works for each of us.

"Besides, it's fun. The more you do it, the more fun it is. It provides a very intimate way to connect with our clients. This brings a lot of joy to me personally as a nurse.

"Many nurses would like to find tools to make them feel better and enjoy their work more. This work does that; it keeps it fresh and exciting. I feel very fortunate to be able to work with people in this way. It is a tool that can go along with the technology. It doesn't have to be used instead of medicine, it can be used as an adjunct."

Lisa's Healing Adventure

"I've been a pediatric nurse for ten years, specializing in inpatient oncology and hematology. After three years of doing that and burning out, I switched to being a nurse clinician in pediatric endocrinology, metabolism, and nutrition. I was also an assistant head nurse in a general pediatrics unit for a year because the hours were more convenient while I was in school.

"I have always used some form of imagery with the children to provide relaxation. With older kids, I liked to 'take them to the beach.' I now realize that I could have also used it to help their parents relax as well.

"I find this imagery work so important, and I believe that most nurses do it instinctively. We forget that the little distractions we use in working with children are really imagery. When we give them opportunities to expand their creative imagination, it can be amazing.

"For example, when a nurse is talking to a child about his favorite things to do while the nurse is doing a procedure, it is actually a form of imagery. In the playroom, when children are playing with different toys and acting out their feelings, we always look at it as distraction. Now I see that it is a form of imagery and role playing.

"Four years ago I moved out West from the East coast. I was immediately involved in a car accident in which I injured my neck, shoulder, and arm. I haven't been able to work since. I started reading articles about guided imagery and attended a workshop, and I found it very exciting. I wanted to do imagery in my work, then I realized I needed to do it with myself first.

"I've tried so many different things to heal myself, and they have all helped to open me tremendously. I have found how crucial it is to explore other ideas. I think I've become a better nurse for having had this injury. Mostly what I've come to realize is that as nurses, we must learn to help people relax.

"I became a patient of Susan Ezra who worked with me as I struggled with the pain of my accident. At first, I was so frustrated trying to use imagery on my own. In her office, I could quickly and easily feel myself floating away when I did imagery with her. Then when I got home and tried it on my own I felt awkward.

"It took several weeks before I was able to incorporate this practice into my daily life. I think this is one of the problems nurses have — we don't take the time to do healing on ourselves. I have found that in caring for yourself, you are much more able to help others.

"Working with Susan, it got to the point that I could decrease the pain and need for pain medications for an hour or more at a time. Susan made some tapes for me and in using them I have found great strength.

"I loved having the opportunity to work with a nurse on my personal healing process. She has been a wonderful listener, very supportive. She made me feel that she really cares about me and it feels wonderful. I feel closer to her because I am a nurse and I know she understands.

"I've learned from all this to expect more in my own care. I know how difficult it is to be a charge nurse, but I also know that we have to find that time to be with the person and make a difference in the quality of his experience.

"Because I have been unable to work, I have had to get more creative about making contributions. For two years, I have been assisting in research studies at the School of Nursing (family health care nursing) at UCSF (volunteering). I miss my work so much that this has become part of my therapy. It's perfect because they feel fortunate and I feel fortunate.

"We've been studying children's pain postoperatively as we move them. We are testing a new assessment tool for children and adolescents to identify pain intensity and location. It's a wonderful tool and it should be out very soon. I am delighted to be able to make my contributions creatively.

"Through my accident and the pain I've experienced, I'm not *saying* I'm sympathetic; I truly understand. I have gone through this, and I know what my patients are feeling.

"I'm now seeing a physician who is very open to holistic modalities. She has put me in touch with a support group and has encouraged me to go on with my life, and to make a difference in the ways that I can. She has been very supportive of my imagery approach.

"The accident and the imagery have opened me so much. I've always loved being with children, and I've always had positive responses. Now I feel even closer and more effective. I don't take it personally if I can't connect with all of them, but most of them do seem to know on some deep level that I really do understand.

"My husband has been very supportive of my efforts. He has been curious. He would never do any of these healing modalities, yet I see how stressed he is. I wish he were more open to trying new things; it has made an incredible difference in my life. Now I'm pregnant, and I'm using imagery to contact the baby and enhance my well-being.

"You do have to want to do it all, as it *is* a commitment. I used to worry about whether other people supported my ideas; now I know for myself that it works. If other people want to try it, that's fine, and if not, I know that it has been a great help on my healing journey."

Jan Maxwell: Imagery Specialist, RN, and Self-Healer

"I'd like to share a story of my personal healing using imagery. I was diagnosed in December, 1989 as having two large uterine fibroids. The diagnosis was by sonogram, and I was advised by doctors to consider vaginal hysterectomy right away; otherwise, they felt they would need to do abdominal hysterectomy if the fibroids grew more.

"It was around that time that I was enrolled in my studies at the Academy for Guided Imagery. I befriended an acupuncturist in the program, and we agreed to work with each other using imagery.

"When I heard the medical recommendations, my first impulse was, 'No, I'm not doing that yet. I want to give myself every opportunity to use adjunctive care and contribute to my own health.' I was not totally rejecting the recommendations of Western medicine, but I wanted to feel I had done everything possible to avoid unnatural means. I didn't want to sit back and feel like a victim. I was also interested in Chinese medical philosophy, so I asked my acupuncturist friend to work with me.

"We did a number of imagery sessions. I went in to see my nurse practitioner, who was overseeing my case in March. By then, there was no change in size of my tumors. I continued to do herbs, acupuncture, and imagery. In the sessions, I incorporated the beliefs from both Western and Eastern medicine. I knew that Chinese doctors believe fibroids to be caused by stagnation of blood, so I envisioned the blood moving through my body, cleansing my uterus.

"In my imagery sessions, a beautiful energy would come as my inner healer. She was ethereal, with no real facial features, but a strong, calm presence. At one point, a couple of weeks prior to the later visit where no fibroids were found, in my imagery she 'took' my uterus and washed it in the ocean's surf. It was a beautiful, very feminine experience, with the surf, the moon, the ocean and its tides. It all felt very cleansing. I used that image a lot in future sessions.

"In all, we did more than a dozen sessions to work with my inner healer. After a few months, I had a very powerful imagery session in which my inner healer told me I didn't need those fibroids anymore. I was truly almost afraid to believe they could be gone, but upon visiting the nurse practitioner, she confirmed that they were gone and that my uterus felt wonderful and healthy.

"Not long after, the nurse practitioner moved away, and I went in for an examination by the new woman gynecologist. After examining me, she said, 'You have no evidence of having ever had fibroids.' She honestly did not seem to believe that they had been there, even though I assured her it had been diagnosed by sonogram.

"Imagery is the facilitator of the healing process. It gets us back to remembering that that's what all this technology is about. We're helping people to heal on very deep levels."

Claramae Weber, RN, Creative Visualizer

"To me, creative visualization is the art of using your imagination to create what you want in your life. I came to realize that I have been using this skill as long as I could remember.

"One of my earliest memories is at age three. I had suffered an injury to my left arm and was in Children's Hospital in Pittsburgh. As I lay in my crib bed, I was cared for by nurses who also sang and laughed with me. I recall at that time seeing a picture in my mind of myself dressed as one of those people in white clothes. I knew right then and there that I wanted to be a nurse. It remained a clear picture, guiding me to enter nursing school at age eighteen.

"At age five I discovered that I had the ability to fly around in my mind and look down at the events of my world. I could actually go to the park and swing on the swings, but in my mind I was flying to China. At that time, I was reading a book about a young girl in China and while I read, I envisioned myself standing with that girl on the Great Wall of China.

"I also had an imaginary friend, Leah. She added so much fun to my life. She was ethereal with blonde hair, blue eyes and beautiful aqua gowns, and she wore sparkling shoes. She and I would dream together and I would tell her my adventures. She would encourage me to great heights of imagination, and she told me that one day I would do all I had dreamed about.

"In my family, however, daydreaming and imagining were not allowed. In fact, they often led to threats or punishment. Needless to say, I tucked all my imagining away to a very hidden place! Unknown to anyone, however, I continued to 'fly around the world' in my mind. My imagination always got me through.

"All the transformational events in my life were preceded by imagining and knowing ahead of time. I knew I had a special sensitivity to people and events. I knew who I would marry long before we ever dated. I knew when I would have children. I now have two wonderful sons and a wonderful daughter who all have great gifts of intelligence, intuition, and imagination.

"When I started as a nurse, I went into psychiatry. I figured I could find out who I was through this work. I did learn a lot, thanks to all my patients for their teachings about abnormal behavior. What wondrous years!

"Things went well for me until my mother died. I went into a tailspin of depression and cried every day for a year. We had been living out of the country from 1966 to 1979, and it felt as if my wonderful life had ended at forty. What a dark night of the soul! The next few years I was mentally 'at sea.' My children and husband were miserable, and we were a very dysfunctional family.

"Eventually, one of the people I worked with told me about a woman by the name of Shakti Gawain, who taught the process called creative visualization. A light went on in my head, my imagination returned, and I knew I had to meet her. From 1981 to 1984, I attended everything she did initially and had a private session once a week. My mental health returned and I flourished. Imagery became my healer.

"In 1984, Shakti invited me to work for her. I became her workshop coordinator and was her workshop assistant until 1988. I then knew I understood the process and wanted to teach it myself, and did so from 1988 to 1992. I had regained the ability to use my imagination that I had discovered at age five. Now I knew what to do with it and was able to share this with others.

"For the past five years, I have been active in the American Holistic Nurses Association. I love this group of dynamic, creative, imaginative, intuitive people. I am now considered a Holistic Nurse and a Healing Touch practitioner and instructor. Through a great many workshops and private sessions, I have learned that for me, imagery is not just a process, it is who I am. Now I reach an even larger audience by teaching other nurses.

"My vision for the future is to take all of this into parish nursing, consulting, and teaching the religious community how to use these spiritual gifts of imagination and intuition. I have been traveling to the West Indies these past six years and have established myself as a healer, teacher, and creativity consultant in Trinidad.

"Recently, an opportunity to be part of a healing center has presented itself. I will be exploring the path as to how to get there when the time is ready. My husband continues to support my work.

"This is a time of great transformation on this planet. We are divine expressions of the creative principle. Now is the time to prove the supremacy of the imagination and intuition in our own lives. We have the tools. They are our thoughts, our will, our purposes, our convictions, and our determination.

"I will always love the little five-year-old girl who lives inside me, along with Leah, my imaginary childhood friend. They guide and direct me today. What fun it is to be using imagination as a nurse during this special time!"

Anna Keck, RN, Nurse Practitioner, Self-Healer

"I've been a nurse practitioner since 1975, and have been in my own practice, Wellcare Associates, since 1983. I have a long history of using imagery, relaxation, and counseling in my work. My practice focuses on illness as a metaphor for growth and spiritual development. My encounter with breast cancer gave me the opportunity to 'walk my talk.'

"I had been having regular mammograms every two years, and had no risk factors except the obvious one of being a woman. I have no family history of cancer, nursed my children, and had a very healthy diet. I felt risk-factor free.

"That's why it was so shocking when I was diagnosed with breast cancer in 1991. I noticed a lump in my breast eight months prior to the diagnosis, and had a mammogram, which was negative. Falsely reassured, I worked with acupuncture and homeopathy as part of my healing program. I had been denied insurance coverage by three different companies because I was in private practice as a nurse practitioner. (This actually became one of my miracles; after I was diagnosed, I eventually received medical insurance only because the state of California had just created a program called 'major risk,' funded through cigarette taxation, for anyone who has been denied insurance within the last year and can prove it, and subsequently develops a life-threatening disease. This program miraculously came into effect one month prior to my diagnosis, however, I had to fight to qualify during chemotherapy.)

"Two weeks after the initial diagnosis, I was struggling with serious decisions and very little information. I had to choose whether to do lumpectomy versus mastectomy; at that time, all I knew was the type of cancer they had identified. I asked a trusted colleague to do an imagery session with me.

"The following is from a journal entry I recorded about that session:

'I asked for clarity, for the one who knows, so I might know what to choose.

'My deep relaxation allows me to descend; I walk down five steps of light; I step off onto a path, leading me to a green mountain top. I emerge, younger in form and energy; the embodiment of spring. My dress is gossamer white, arms are outstretched behind me, opening my chest.

'I embrace the sunlight, and it pours into my chest. My guide invites me to bring the light into my chest. The image is powerful; there is a light, shadowy energy under my arm. Suddenly I experience a rapid energy shift, as if water jets are expelling all the breast contents (under force), leaving only skin and nipple.

'I am completely cleaned out, leaving fresh tissue. A gremlin appears. He is irreverently wearing the nipple as a hat. Even though I'm in a trance, I smile and ask him why he is so flippant with my breast.

'He says I need to lighten up. He then goes to my axilla and repeats the cleansing. He cleans my armpit, then goes off in a pixie-like fashion, eventually resting in a crescent moon in my armpit. I am so tired and relaxed I can't move, except to stroke my armpit and breast.

'Then I am guided to go to the water, where I see my reflection both in my youth and in the present. I begin to cry and cry, then I take off my clothes and get into the water. I let it cleanse me, then I go onto the rocks to rest naked.

'Suddenly the rock changes and under me I feel something that feels like a large and furry animal. I'm wondering if it is a horse or a dog. I realize it is a bear, with a coat so thick and furry it reminds me of my dog Alex. The fur is white, like a polar bear (which has been my guide in previous imagery sessions). This time I sense him kinesthetically; his coat isn't visible until I've been lifted and carried by him.'

"As regards the eventual outcome, when I had surgery, the margins were clean, lymph nodes were negative. They got all the cancer with only a lumpectomy, as the cancer had not spread. A major gift was that I went into surgery feeling completely confident and relaxed. After the session I could now trust my breasts and body to be cancer free. I could trust myself to have a lumpectomy and to thrive.

"In my subsequent work, I've been in contact with Caryle Hirshberg (1993), who wrote a book for the Institute of Noetic Science about spontaneous remission. She informed me that the gremlin is one of the universal symbols, a worldwide image in art and imagery from cultures around the world. It was validation of the deep aspects of our healing mind.

"Caryle identifies several behaviors and attitudes for long-term survival:

1. It has been found that *acceptance* increases immune function (whereas fatalism decreases immunity).

2. It is important to have a collaborative relationship with your doctor. Be sure to shop until you find the right one to work with.

3. It is valuable to live each day as if it is precious.

4. Breaking isolation, asking for help from others, is important.

5. It is important to find ways to actively and appropriately manage fear and anxiety.

6. Make the decision to live for yourself and think 'If I'm going to die, I'll do it *my* way!'

"Caryle also identifies five characteristics of long-term survivors and spontaneous remitters; these traits often don't show up until the person is challenged. Long-term survivors and spontaneous remitters:

1. accept the disease and diagnosis; denial only works when it is absolute, which is infrequent. They maintain a fighting spirit.

2. are true to themselves.

3. don't accept what they used to accept without careful examination.

4. eliminate the 'garbage' from their lives.

5. learn to say NO!

"I began to keep a miracle list, because there were so many wonderful things happening that were beyond the realm of the ordinary since my diagnosis. Just as one example, a doctor I had known thirty years earlier when learning of my situation offered to operate at no charge, and I stayed at his house for recovery with a nurse friend of mine whom I also brought in the OR with me. She read a prayer I wrote while I was undergoing anesthesia. I even brought my bear claw into surgery (power symbol), keeping it close to my body. I asked for and got what I wanted.

"As for my advice to nurses: Do your inner work; listen to your own wisdom; remove the obstacles to allowing the incredible universal force to come into you and help you to heal.

"I truly am living the life of my dreams on every level. My process taught me about surrender. I had to let go of my mind trying to figure everything out. When I did, I became much more aligned with the spirit world, and grace poured upon me. I felt like a feather carried by the wind.

"Everyone comes to their place of surrender in their own way. For me it was through reading Larry LeShan's book *Cancer as a Turning Point* (1989). His writing challenged me to consider what it is that inspires me, and reminded me to be true to what I really love. He encouraged me to discover what was unlived in my life and to eliminate those things that stress me. At first it sounded selfish, but I've learned that it is really what self-care is about.

"I try to make the care I give others equal to what I give to myself. My life has completely changed. I'm now in a wonderful relationship (soon to be married), have a beautiful garden, a fruitful practice, and I feel centered and focused. My whole nursing practice reflects this. I am committed to living from my center and everything arises from this space of the heart. I am more thoughtful about what I say yes to.

"Nurses are the change agents for the culture. We are moving toward health care rather than sick care, and we need to care for ourselves."

Terry Miller, RN, MS, Imagery Consultant

"I attended a holistic nursing workshop years ago called the 'Turning Point.' It was there that I began to recognize how pivotal nursing is in being a catalyst for healing, and how much of a relationship there is between the body, mind, and spirit.

"As an intensive care nurse, I suddenly realized how important high touch is to high tech. I saw that there is so much more than symptoms, and I began to feel that I was missing a lot by focusing primarily on the physical component.

"I also became aware that an educational process could really touch nurses once they sat down to hear it. I decided that I wanted to teach the 'Turning Point,' because it literally took me out of burnout as a director of an intensive care unit. What a relief! I no longer had the burden of thinking I had to fix everything.

"It took me a year to incorporate changing my own lifestyle. I spent that year working on prevention, examining how I thought, and what I believed. Then I started teaching the 'Turning Point,' about holistic principles, death, and dying. It was around that time that I heard about the Academy for Guided Imagery. Doctors Marty Rossman and David Bresler were teaching professionals how to incorporate body-mind principles in the clinical setting.

"I quit my position as a nursing unit director, and soon left the intensive care unit. After a period of equilibration I enrolled in the Certificate Program at the Academy for Guided Imagery, followed by another year, and became a faculty member.

"It was there that Sue, Jan, and I birthed the 'Beyond Ordinary Nursing' workshop. We all realized that the balance was very important, that to be a healer one must first apply principles of the bodmind with oneself.

"We saw that when one is doing healing work, you are not the healer, you are the catalyst. Your job is to hold the space for others to heal.

"Imagery is my heartwork. It helps me in everything I do. I not only use imagery with clients, I seek my own imagery experiences with colleagues to resolve my personal and professional issues.

"I find it very healing to be in that sacred space, of truly and wholeheartedly listening to someone else. In this manner, I am very present to that person, and not interpreting, as I used to do in traditional nursing.

"Doing the work teaches me to honor people as they are, not to fix them. It is my lifework, not only my avocation; it is my mission. I envision myself continuing my private practice into my ninth decade. I learned imagery from others; now I can pass it on and help them move into their own healing by holding the space.

"Imagery is invaluable not only in helping me to be present, but in my personal life as well. For example, when I am feeling conflicted, I will resort to parts work. I will engage the part of me that wants to do something versus the part of me that resists. I often ask if I really want to continue working part-time in a hospital, and to gain clarity, I contact the part that wants to stay and the part that wants to leave.

"Similarly, if I find myself anxious, working with highly stressed people, I use imagery rehearsal, asking myself such questions as 'How do I want to come across?' or "How would I like to feel?'

"I check in with my inner advisor before I make any big decisions. In this way, I have learned to honor the gut reactions of my intuitive self. I would use it to decide about a change in job position, or other decisions. In doing this, I learn to honor that emotional part of myself, and to trust that part of me that already knows the answers for my life.

"Imagery is a great leveler for nurses, not only in learning how to help the patient, but also in helping ourselves to be balanced and healthy. When you do this work, you are healing yourself *and* healing others simultaneously. I can't think of a better position to be in!

"To other nurses, I would say that having a broad perspective is everything. Never say 'never,' or choose to believe that things won't work out. Refuse to look at things simply on the scientific plane; keep everything open to what might be possible. Remember, the world was once thought to be flat; now we know differently. Be open.

"If nurses can get in touch with their inner wisdom, learn to trust their own feelings and instincts, they will achieve a sense of balance. Getting in touch also takes away compulsiveness and self-esteem issues. It further helps nurses to be present to themselves and others. It prevents burnout. Imagery makes things exciting, helps you see the big picture.

"As a final thought, it is not in changing the things outside that makes a difference; it's how you choose to look at things from inside out."

SUMMARY

We can learn from these imaginative nurses how much potential really exists for creating our lives as we would like them to be. With models such as these, it becomes easier for us to envision ourselves making the necessary changes that will enable us to take a powerful position in the emerging health care model and to enjoy our nursing endeavors.

References

Hirshberg, C. (1993). *Spontaneous remission: An annotated bibliography.* Sausalito, CA: Institute of Noetic Sciences.

LeShan, L. (1989). *Cancer as a turning point.* New York: E.P. Dutton.

Yogananda, P. (1946). *The autobiography of a yogi.* Los Angeles: Self Realization Fellowship.

NURSE, HEAL THYSELF: BEGINNING THE JOURNEY

Every nurse must begin the personal and professional journey toward feeling whole to become part of a powerful solution together.

Karilee Halo Shames, 1993

In beginning to provide a viable model for health enhancement, nurses must become living examples of that which we propose for our patients. This chapter introduces some early steps for nurses who wish to become models for their patients and be believable teachers of health. It then discusses how nurses can begin to practice and incorporate imagery techniques into their daily personal and professional lives.

WHERE TO BEGIN: INITIAL STEPS FOR NURSES

Codependence Issues

The first issue that must be addressed for nurses to become healthy models is the topic of codependency. In listening to nurses' stories, one often hears that the nurse was attracted to her work because someone in the family needed help and nurturing when the nurse was young. Many nurses have been taking care of others their entire lives. Some authors writing about nursing and codependency assert that more than 83 percent of people in the helping professions come from dysfunctional families.

It is difficult to prove or disprove such statistics. Many nurses vehemently deny having grown up in a chaotic household. Certainly one thing is apparent: how we choose to view our experiences is a very personal issue. What might feel dreadful and abusive to one person might feel fine to another. Nonetheless, it does seem to be common that people in the nursing profession always wanted to help, to make a difference; perhaps they gave much more than they received in their efforts to feel useful.

These traits should not be viewed as negative. It is not helpful to judge the ways people choose to live. What seems most important is that we learn to honor each other for our unique journeys and the marvelous ways we have learned to transform that which was painful into something meaningful and helpful for humankind. In honoring our special gifts, nursing can most quickly rise to acquire the public's trust.

In exploring codependency, we are asked to examine our learned behavior. We must decide if the coping defenses we established years ago are still helpful. In looking clearly at our patterns, we are often able to see that we may have been operating on automatic pilot, without really making conscious decisions about what is true and helpful for us today.

CASE STUDY | *Mary, the ER Nurse*

Consider the example of Mary, an ER nurse in the Midwest, who is 32 years old and weighs 240 pounds. Mary was the oldest of eight children. Her father died when she was thirteen, and she had to work alongside her mother for many years, raising the remaining children and helping to support her mother.

Mary never married or dated much. She entered nursing school immediately after high school, working long hours in part-time positions to bring in money. She has been depressed for many years, occasionally taking strong antidepressant drugs to help her battle mental fatigue.

Though she is now a head nurse on the day shift, she has little joy in her life. She lacks the respect of her peers, many of whom find her bitter and difficult to please. They also view her as humorless, and they occasionally play childish pranks to lighten the mood on the unit. Mary has a difficult time sharing anger, and she fluctuates between losing her temper and being overly nice in the face of great pressure.

All this takes its toll on Mary, and she leaves the unit exhausted. She goes home, unable to find the energy for any social life whatsoever. Even the simple tasks of self care, such as food shopping, cleaning, and laundry feel overwhelming to her.

In considering Mary's plight, we can readily see that Mary seems to feel trapped. She exhibits no creativity or enjoyment, and she seems to be going through the motions of her life without really living. This is a classic example of the ravages of codependency.

When we are living in a codependent state, we often operate on automatic pilot. The programs that play out in our behaviors are frequently those we learned as children to cope with the demands of our young lives.

Unfortunately, these patterns become ingrained habits, chaining us to lifestyles that may have nothing to do with the adult lives we have managed to create. In

Mary's case, she learned so well to care for others and neglect her own needs that she lives presently as if she had no needs.

In reality, Mary needs to take a good look at her life and make some different decisions. She needs to reconsider her working patterns in relation to the life she wants for herself. She must no longer take care of a large group of people. In fact, Mary lives alone and could easily create a much more enjoyable existence. She could make new decisions and free herself for more self-care. The addition of some simple self-healing maneuvers would greatly enhance the quality of Mary's existence.

Reprogramming: Enhancing Life Quality

There are several steps one must take to begin to enjoy life more fully. If nurses are to be able to help others take this journey, they must first travel on their own self-healing paths. In this way, nurses become more competent guides on the healing journey.

First, to improve the quality of one's existence, one must recognize that a problem exists. The codependent nurse operates on automatic. She has been unwilling to take a good look at her life, so she is unaware of the many ways in which her needs are not being met. She might yearn for something different, but does not know how to find it. She usually considers that the solution to her problems, and the cause, lie outside of herself. Herein begins her challenge; she must redirect the focus to look within, both for causation and cure.

Second, the nurse might analyze some of her prime operating beliefs. Our beliefs are often the driving force behind ingrained behavioral patterns. If we are to heal the unhealthy habits, we must be willing to look beyond the behavior and consider why we chose to act in that manner. For this reason, most people in the healing professions seek outside professional help at some point or other.

It is very difficult to see our patterns; in fact, many people do not see their behavior as patterns. They consider the ways they act as descriptions of who they are. The reality is that the behavior is not necessarily who the person is, but is a reflection of the life he has lived, combined with the coping mechanisms he developed to survive that life.

To find out who one really is, one must release the dysfunctional patterns and explore. This is a necessary part of the healing journey, and it often requires the support of others who have traveled similar paths. In this manner, we become guides for each other, and ultimately for our patients.

You might want to read some of the introductory or comprehensive books listed in the Appendix. There are a great many well-written volumes about imagery and the process of self-healing. You may also enjoy browsing through catalogs and reviews. In addition, many of the most popular books are now out on tape.

CREATIVE IMAGININGS

As you can now see, there are indeed many creative ways to use the power of the mind. Ancient peoples learned to harness this power to ward off evil. In today's more complex and sophisticated world, nurses and healers must learn to keep the mind strong and not be easily influenced by others.

In his best-selling motivational book *Think and Grow Rich*, Napoleon Hill (1960) stressed the idea that one main element separating those people who are successful from those who are not is the ability to avoid the negative influence of others.

Changing-the-Mind Channel

As healers, when we learn to use the mind for self-preservation, we can convey that ability to those entrusted to our care. One simple technique to demonstrate this ability is what I call "changing-the-mind channel."

When involved in a situation where there is considerable negative or disruptive influence, just imagine making your best decision about how to handle that situation. Then see yourself following your plan, regardless of any offensive comments or maneuvers against it. Strong leaders must be prepared to face some adversity and opposition. This is best accomplished by knowing that you will follow through with your plan and will not allow the negative thought patterns of others to distract you from your mission. This is a simple technique for finding inner strength when one must face and overcome adversity.

Visual Affirmation

Another concept I have coined is the idea of a *visual affirmation.* This refers to the use of imagery to create a positive picture of the future, with the intent to reinforce this image and inspire its occurrence in real life. As an example, if I wanted to spend a relaxing weeklong vacation with my family in Hawaii this summer, I might begin by picturing us there, having a wonderful time reading and relaxing, playing in the gentle ocean waves and feeling peaceful and joyful.

I can picture this desired event over and over, many times a day, perhaps enhancing the image with smells, sounds, and feelings that would accompany this scene. While this is actually a positive rehearsal, it is more a creation of an affective state than an action. It is not a matter of accomplishing some specific activity, as in the case of many athletes who use positive rehearsal. Rather, I see it as a chance to affirm my deepest desires by imagining that it has already happened and by enjoying the feelings I will be feeling when this scene actually occurs.

Yet another process I have found very helpful in working with patients is what could be called *software replacement imagery,* a technique that has been mentioned previously. In this technique, the client is encouraged to examine his behavioral or emotional programs as if they could be viewed on a computer screen. When he recognizes programs that are reactions to earlier life traumas, and that may no longer serve his healthiest needs, the client can make a mental decision to take that program out of the mental computer and replace it with something much more positive and life-affirming.

For instance, suppose a nurse is talking to Susie, a college student who has some medical problems that are compounded by the stress of recalling earlier painful childhood experiences. Susie would like to have a healthy relationship with a man, but she was heavily abused by her father. Because of these difficult early experiences, Susie learned to fear men. Now, however, Susie can be encouraged to relax, close her eyes, and see a computer screen. Next, she imagines a folder on the computer screen called "male abuse." She can then envision that she is dumping that program. In its place, Susie creates a file called "healthy male relationships." Now she is up and running with a new program.

Imagine the enormous power of being able to throw your old programs into the garbage and watch while they are gobbled up. A person might use this type of imagery to assist with a variety of difficult aspects of his life. It is often helpful for a person to picture his life as if it were the desktop on a computer. He might see different folders, representing the various components of his life, across the desktop. As he clicks on certain folders, he might notice old programs flashing before him, some of which are very uncomfortable.

Most of us carry old programs mentally, wearing them on our bodies and in our psyches. We get plugged in to our old wounding, act in distorted manners, and don't seem to know how to stop running these hurtful mental scenes.

Dumping the Rubbish

You might try this exercise for yourself at this point. Imagine your life folders flashing across the screen in your mind's eye. Watch as you open any of these folders and see some painful old program before your eyes. Notice your bodily response; pay attention to any emotions or feelings at this time.

Now take that folder and drag it toward the garbage. How are you feeling as this occurs? For some people, the change cannot happen too quickly, while others take time to let go. Each of us has our own pace for creating and accepting change. Learn to honor your needs as you embark upon your self-healing journey. Learn to listen to your emotions and intuition as you prepare to make changes.

You will begin to see how creative a task it is to heal yourself. This is a very exciting prospect, and you may find yourself feeling a bit shaky. Keep in mind that all change is scary and exciting at the same time. When you see how alive you feel, you will begin to experience the joy that arises from living in truth and integrity. The process is something that will enrich all the work you do and will begin to prepare you for the role of nurse-healer.

Decisional Affirmation

The previous process goes hand-in-hand with another one called *decisional affirmation.* In this process, the client is encouraged to make a commitment about how he intends to live his life, then to use that image as a guiding light in daily decisions. The way to think about this process is that the commitment becomes a rudder that steers life forward in a positive direction. Whenever it is time to make another decision, the decision is made by rescrutinizing the major commitment to see if it is in alignment with the highest priorities.

I often encourage clients and nurses to take time to get in touch with their soul's purpose. This gives the person a chance to decide actively the reason he feels he is here. When people are on their personal paths to healing, and are aligned with their unique purposes, they are much healthier and effective.

According to many ancient cultures, including Native-American tradition, every person is a piece of the "Great Mystery." Each of us has a special piece of the puzzle of life, which makes us equally unique and valuable.

In getting to the core of our life purpose, we cut away much of the "dead wood," that which no longer serves as we take the most growthful path. When we choose to align with our soul's highest purpose and continue to regularly affirm the image of ourselves in our most powerful roles, we have created decisional affirmations. Each time we choose to honor our life goals, we have affirmed those goals through our decisions, thus strengthening our commitment.

Similarly, another kind of decisional process is when a patient has made a decision on some level that life is not worth living and that he would be better off dead.

We nurses often see people in our work who seem to have given up. Unless we can reach the person's soul and inspire its connection with purpose, the person often chooses to lose faith and give up on life. High-level nursing is often able to touch a person in such a deep way that he can change that view of himself, deciding to live more productively and fully. The decision is always his.

WHOLE-PERSON NURSING CARE

Our work is most meaningful when we empower our clients to do their own healing work. We must learn to honor their decisions, rather than to try to impose our will on them. This is not to say that we don't try to support clients in finding their places of peace, and in making choices that support the highest good, but we must become more and more clear about the boundaries of healthy relationship if we are to survive and thrive as professionals.

Setting Boundaries

There are many ways nurses can learn to strengthen their boundaries for healthier relationships with patients and peers. Some of these can be approached as fun and joyful imagery exercises.

One of the most powerful exercises is to imagine yourself protected inside a bubble. This bubble can extend as far as you need it to to feel comfortable and safe. You might wish to create your bubble to meet your needs.

I find it helpful to imagine that the bubble is made of a semipermeable membrane. This membrane allows the small light molecules (i.e., love, appreciation) to pass through, yet screens out the larger, more dense molecules (negativity, criticalness, lack of support).

Nurses often work under very difficult circumstances. Hospital environments have not always been designed with the health of staff in mind. In the days of Florence Nightingale, considerable thought was given to the architectural creation in terms of fresh air, light, and sound. Today, health care facilities do not seem to reflect the same concern for employees or patients.

The nurse who stays healthy and learns to protect herself from stale thoughts and stale energies becomes a model for others. She also feels better more of the time and inspires others to take better care of themselves.

More and more, we see the birth of exercise facilities in close proximity to health care facilities. Nurses must learn to take the time to revitalize, and they can also learn simultaneously to protect themselves from negativity within the environment.

Negativity can arise from physical or mental causation. When nurses work together in close proximity, and dishonor each other through negative thoughts and deeds, there is a poison that spreads through the unit. On the other hand, when nurses support and honor each other, that positive energy flows into the unit as well, causing ripples of harmony to flood the area. We all know the difference in feeling between these two environments.

Napoleon Hill (1960) made some interesting comments about what *intuition* truly is. According to *Think and Grow Rich*, Hill writes that intuition arises when all the senses are finely attuned. There is a synergy created when this happens, so that we can sense more subtle energies. When we are truly seeing, hearing, tasting, smelling, and feeling, we inspire a high level of attunement, one that allows for receipt of more subtle information from the environment.

This special gift, one of nursing's greatest strengths, can also work against us if we are not selective about our input. If we are open to all levels of information, and the feeling tone in our surroundings is hostile, we can become damaged and weakened. For these reasons, it is crucial that nurses learn to screen information and to set boundaries in a way that maximizes their senses of well-being.

Another way to empower oneself with boundaries is through the use of clear, assertive communication. Many people find that they are able to communicate what they mean to say most clearly when they picture what it is they want first. In this way, imagery becomes a very powerful ally for the nurse in her professional endeavors.

Napoleon Hill (1960) also felt that all great achievements begin with an idea. An idea often arrives in the form of a positive picture. If the nurse has a particularly challenging patient, she might imagine what she needs to do by picturing what might happen in her mind.

This process is often compared to the viewing of a movie. We can consider our minds a blank screen across which we project images that correspond to our thoughts or desires. At times, we can figure out what we need to do by imaging the scene in the future.

Not everyone sees in picture form, but all of us perceive sensations that guide us in our lives. Some people might feel uncomfortable when contemplating a particular scenario. Others might recall a similar event with positive, or disastrous, results. The mind is infinitely creative in its ability to conjure images, and part of our healing comes from connecting with our inner processes and learning from within ourselves.

Accessing Inner Guidance for Nursing

One nurse, Georgia, tells the story of working with a particularly difficult patient who had multiple sclerosis. The woman, Ms. Smith, had been diagnosed recently, and was terrified about the implications this disease had for her life. She was accustomed to being in control, and she was unable to verbalize her fear and sense of vulnerability. Instead, she chose to bark orders irritably at the staff, occasionally using profane language and raising her voice so it reverberated through the halls.

Many of the nurses had tried to cooperate with Ms. Smith to no avail. She was unpleasant despite how someone interacted with her. The staff were frustrated and angry.

After several days, Georgia went in to work with Ms. Smith and was practically thrown out of the room. Rather than leave, however,

Georgia chose to seek a solution. She decided to take a few moments in quiet reflection in the linen room to gather her thoughts and consult her inner guidance for a deeper level of wisdom about this situation.

After a minute or two, she had an image of a shy little girl who was terrified and afraid to ask for help. She felt extremely tender toward this child and asked the child mentally if she needed some help. The child nodded tearfully, and reached out her hand. In her mind, Georgia took her hand, held it in her own, and offered soothing words in a soft, melodic voice. At first, the child remained frozen, but gradually she seemed to melt in the warmth of the tenderness. After a while, the child moved in closer, and soon the two were hugging.

Georgia made the decision to appeal to Ms. Smith's inner child, who was obviously terrified. All efforts to support the woman were rejected, yet Georgia felt certain that there was a way to make headway with this patient.

Georgia returned to the room, moving slowly and cautiously. In her mind, she held the image of Ms. Smith as a frightened young child. She had decided to never waver from this view of Ms. Smith, no matter how intimidating she appeared.

When Ms. Smith barked at Georgia, Georgia spoke softly and firmly. "Ms. Smith, if I were in your position, I think I would feel very scared. I have thought about what this must all feel like to you, and I imagine it is very lonely. I would like for you to feel better. Would it be all right with you if I took your hand for a minute? (Ms. Smith nodded.) Just for a minute, imagine that I am someone who knows you very well and really cares about your well-being. Who might I be?"

At this point, a small voice came from the patient. "My Aunt Rose. She was the only one who knew me. Everyone else just treated me as someone to take for granted and make assumptions about. No one seemed to care about getting to know how I really felt."

Notice how the interchange has shifted. The nurse was able to find a way into the patient's reality. There was nothing exceptional or magical about her approach. The only thing she really did differently was to access her inner wisdom in her efforts to seek guidance that would be useful in this situation. She trusted her inner information enough to act on it without having to interpret and fully understand it.

Georgia was able to break through barriers because she did not accept past behaviors as self-limiting. She has obviously worked with imagery enough to be able and willing to listen to the images and honor whatever message she receives from them. This is not a difficult process; in fact, it is quite simple and useful to nurses. There are many ways in which we receive direction, and we might consider being open to utilizing them all for the benefit of our own health and our patient care.

Setting Boundaries with Clear Communications

Another way nurses can protect themselves and empower patients is through clear communication. Many of nursing's challenges arise from the overly aggressive or passive-aggressive models of communications we exhibit.

The major difference between aggression and assertion is that in assertion we are able to get our needs met without taking away from anyone else. Aggression has been explained as getting what one desires by stepping on someone else.

In promoting assertive communications, once again we can consult with our inner wisdom to gain a clear picture of what it is we hope to accomplish. Once we are able to see it, or feel it, or sense what it feels like, we can allow our communications to flow from this place of knowing so that we can achieve our desires.

Choices in Communication

Consider the example of the nurse who wishes to have a particular weekend off, and who has an "indirectly aggressive" manager. Mary asked for next weekend off months ago, but her manager, Sharon, has never directly agreed to Mary's request.

Mary has a cousin who is getting married that weekend and she must know today. She is feeling irritated and unacknowledged. She is prepared to tell Sharon in no uncertain terms how she feels and what she thinks, whether it costs her her job or not.

Mary decides, however, to consult with Lucy (another nurse) first about how she might handle this situation. Lucy is known for her ease in communicating and in helping to clarify situations without hurting anyone's feelings.

Lucy listens to Mary's story, then suggests that Mary take a minute to relax and travel to a place that feels safe and comfortable to her. In this special place, Mary is to meet with her Inner Advisor, asking how to best handle the situation so it can result in everyone feeling good.

The guide tells Mary that she is angry because this situation does not feel new to her. Mary has often been in this position before. She is initially advised to separate the earlier experiences from the present one. Then, when she can see it more clearly for what it is, she can find the words that will enable her to convey her desire without getting caught in the potential trap that has been laid for her. She will have learned from past experience.

Mary recognizes that in her early life she felt very unheard. She was the invisible one, the one who tried not to make waves because there was already so much turmoil. She learned to be docile and to do without rather than to ask for what she wanted.

In seeing this, Mary recognizes the opportunity presented to her in this situation. Her attitude shifts. She no longer feels it a burden to have to talk to Sharon; instead, it becomes a chance to do things in a new way. This is a learning experience.

Mary feels better about the task at hand. With this attitude, she asks Sharon when might be a good time to take a few minutes with her. Sharon looks surprised, but responds appropriately.

By the time they meet, Mary has already decided several things she is going to try to do differently. She starts by making herself comfortable and positions herself physically so as to be equal with Sharon. She has also determined that this time off is something she needs and deserves; therefore, she is much more positive about the likelihood of being granted what she asks. Her attitude is positive and upbeat.

She has also decided to speak from a position of power. She has gathered the facts, and she knows who is available during that time, so she can ask for what she wants.

Because many of these behaviors are not characteristic of Mary's previous dealings, Sharon is not prepared for Mary to hold her ground so well; thus Mary has an advantage. Also, Mary practiced some imagery rehearsal techniques, and she has already shown Lucy how she would present her case and receive feedback.

Needless to say, by the time all is said and done, Mary and Sharon have reached agreement easily, and each respects the other more for having met as equals. Both feel positive about the results. Mary feels elated, for not only has she accomplished her initial present goal, but in the process she has managed to break some very old patterns, and she feels that this is a new beginning for her. She imagines great possibilities for future undertakings, and she will move ahead quickly in her endeavors.

HELPFUL HINTS

Keep in mind that nurses who wish to incorporate these tools do not have to be perfect in using them to start. All success begins with an idea, and if you can imagine yourself beginning to accomplish your goals, you are on your way to maximizing your efforts.

Do not hesitate to start with your goal in mind, but practice first in more comfortable and secure surroundings before treading on thinner ice. If you are practicing to be more assertive, start with someone you trust and respect to increase your potential for initial successes. Later, you can build on those successes when you have developed greater confidence.

Everyone has to start somewhere, and there are many instructional tools to support your journey. A failure is only deemed such in the view of the person judging, so allow yourself to grow and learn without being harsh on yourself. We can always improve our skills, and we learn to do that through effort and plenty of practice.

SUMMARY

It cannot be said too often: never underestimate the power of the mind. The mind is like a computer. We can take our proper place as its programmer, or we can allow it to run wild. Our work as nurses requires that we move from a centered, calm place. When we act from that place of strength, we make the best decisions and feel better about our lives.

References

Hill, N. (1960). *Think and grow rich.* New York: Ballantine Books/Napoleon Hill Foundation.

Shames, K. (1993). *The nightingale conspiracy: Nursing comes to power in the 21st century.* New York: Enlightenment Press.

WEAVING THE HEALING WEB: INITIAL STEPS, REASSURANCE, AND HELPFUL HINTS

Spider is the female energy of the creative force that weaves the beautiful designs of life . . .

David Carson & Jamie Sams, 1988

As nurses begin to heal themselves and become models for their clients, they also become models for other providers in the health care system. We might consider this network a healing web, such as is made by a spider. The web continues to expand outward, catching others as they curiously explore.

NURSES: WEAVING THE HEALING WEB

In a positive sense, this kind of weaving can be extremely enjoyable and productive. *Healing* is a very comprehensive term, relating to the wholeness of any situation. It is not a thorough healing just because the patient begins to feel better physically. In the deepest levels of healing, all involved receive benefits and are transformed through the process, both inside and out.

Using the imagery of the healing web, we can picture a spider busily spinning her dreams into a pattern. In Native-American tradition, the spider signifies creativity and the need to be productive. As nurses, we need to be more like the spider. We must learn to unleash the tremendous creativity within and enable ourselves to be more creatively productive. However, we must be cautious about the webs in which we might find ourselves entangled! Nursing is a delicate art. Florence Nightingale said it could almost be called the finest of the fine arts.

Many nurses have learned, some the hard way, that nursing can be strenuous mentally, emotionally, and physically. Many nurses have become entangled in webs woven by other nurses who have left some twisted and confused patterns. To be healthy, and effective as a nurse, one must be wary and tread delicately.

As nursing grows and expands, it becomes evident that each of us can contribute to this great professional endeavor. We can learn to use imagery and ritual to enhance our work and our lives, and to expand the healing web outward, encompassing all whose lives we touch.

Nurse-Weaving: Introducing Imagery to Colleagues

As nurses become more comfortable using some of the many techniques described, they may find themselves becoming teachers of this subtle form of healing.

Example: Introducing Imagery to Doctors

As an example, consider the following story as shared by Susan Ezra, Jan Maxwell, and Terry Miller. Jenny is the patient of Dr. Quark. She is three days post op. Nurse Crystal approaches Dr. Quark. The doctor says, "I left an order for pain meds q4h prn; I notice that since you started working with the patient, she has not received any pain medication."

Nurse Crystal responds: "Well, Dr. Quark, Jenny approached me about the possibility of learning some relaxation techniques. I told her that when I had time I would acquaint her with some simple techniques. After I spent a short time with her, she began to try some of the relaxation exercises, and she has not required any pain meds since then!"

Dr. Quark asks Nurse Crystal to prove that these tools are effective, so she cheerfully guides him to several impressive articles in the medical journals. His response? "Er, yes, this looks very interesting."

Nurse-Weaving: Enticing Patients with Imagery

In another scenario, the patient puts his call bell on, and the nurse responds:

Patient: "This pain is awful."

Nurse: "You recently had pain medication."

Patient: "Well, it doesn't seem to be helping. Please, make it go away. I have been so stressed out at work and at home. I can't endure this level of pain any longer."

Nurse: "Would you like to try some relaxation?"

Patient: "How can I relax?"

The nurse proceeds to speak in a soothing tone, allowing the patient to discuss his problems. Before the nurse ever introduces imagery, the patient's anxiety is reduced, because the simple act of listening conveys a sense of concern. Soon the anxiety and pain begin to diminish.

Another way the nurse can introduce the concept to a patient is to role play, as the leaders of the class "Beyond Ordinary Nursing" did for us when they enacted this scene:

An old man, bent over in his chair, called the nurse for something trivial, then spent a few minutes talking with her. She ascertained that much of the man's pain was a result of tremendous anxiety, as his wife was home alone while he was in the nursing home.

The nurse offered to call his wife and tell her some things he wanted her to know, and he began to feel more uplifted. Then the nurse asked if he'd like to try some relaxation. She was able to help him straighten up, and through a simple imagery process, was able to help him find a calm place within. The demands ceased, and the patient now felt that he had a friend.

The nurse could also have pretended to be his wife (role-playing) if the patient needed to talk to his wife about emotional issues and she was unavailable. She could listen as he said all the things he needed to say. In this manner, the patient could imagine that his wife was hearing his anguish, and he could release any anxiety related to his inability to share his feelings.

Weaving Teamwork in the Health Care Environment

Nurses are in an ideal position to promote teamwork in health care. As the intermediary between the patient, the doctor, and ancillary staff, the nurse can truly provide advocacy for the patient and his extended family.

As health care costs escalate, patients are sent home earlier with more acute conditions. Hospitals are reserved for the most acute crisis situations, and families are being asked to carry more and more responsibility for their ailing loved ones. All of these changes result in increased opportunity for nurses to creatively weave networks between people.

There is evidence of a major shift toward nurses as primary providers, and with this shift comes a chance for nurses to view themselves differently. As nurses demonstrate greater respect and honor for each other, the profession advances.

Nursing is a unique and time-honored tradition. Our history is rich with stories of women (and men) who gave up everything they held dear to join convents and devote their lives to the care and feeding of the sick. Whenever plagues struck, nurses came from the ranks of the community to offer loving support to those in need. Today, with the AIDS epidemic, nurses continue to serve in their quiet way, silent heroes amidst a deadly disease.

In San Francisco, the general hospital has devoted a large unit to the care of people challenging AIDS. The nurses have been given free reign on this unit partly because medical science has no cures for this syndrome. There has been tremendous evidence of nurse creativity in this environment, and the nurses seem to truly enjoy their work.

These nurses report learning so much from the patients, many of whom are young and articulate, about what true healing is. Though many of the patients are dying, they feel they have found a new level of peace and contentment in their lives; they feel healed.

The nurses who work under these conditions carry a particular attitude about their work that allows them to transform menial tasks into monumental contributions. Once again, the power of the mind reigns supreme.

Sacred Weavings

Wherever nurses work, there is the potential to weave a sacredness into the environment. In the days of Florence Nightingale, as evidenced in her voluminous writings, much attention was given to the environment. She advised nurses to speak softly, fluff pillows, pay attention to ventilation and lighting. Nurses can consider this attention to fine detail part of the unique and necessary art of nursing. Part of what makes nursing unique is its connection to that which nourishes the spirit and provides beauty.

As nurses grow in the ability to cooperate with each other, we weave new models for healing. Many patients and many nurses are products of less-than-optimal environments in early life. Many of us did not receive the nurturing that supports healthy growth. We went into nursing to find it. It is no wonder that we still fall short of being able to offer that kind of nurturing to our patients, having come from such a lack of modeling.

The perfect antidote is to surround ourselves with positive, nourishing healing energy, so that we and our patients can grow and thrive. The model for this can arise easily from within the ranks of nursing.

The Web Grows

All it takes to reweave the web of nursing is a few nurses with vision who exude a strong and centered type of leadership. Nurses like these become the center of the web, from which other branches are continually woven outward.

They attract others into the web by demonstrating the healing effects of this style. Soon they are surrounded by many others who want to be like them. They even catch those who were nearby in their webs, for the magnetism is strong. They inspire healthy change, and it spreads outward.

Each of us can be the motivating force in weaving a healing web. It takes people of vision to see the far-reaching effects of this kind of modeling behavior. As more of us become involved in presenting healthy models, the evolution from helper to healer becomes faster.

Once we create a loving environment where we work, we can begin to affect all who enter this sacred space. Doctors, family, physical therapists—all these people receive the benefits of a joyful interactive environment. It becomes a place for people to grow and change. There is support for healthier living in this setting, and the old ways die quickly.

In this healthy, nurturing setting, ideally everyone changes. People are willing to try new ideas, take risks, be bold in creating new avenues for expression. Many nurses have reported that even the doctors seem very open and responsive when the environment is conducive to healthy change.

Doctors and Nurses

The doctor-nurse relationship is another aspect in need of healing. A running competition between doctors and nurses seems to exist, with each side vying for more power. It is naive to believe we can carry on competitive relationships within health facilities and expect people to receive optimal care.

We nurses can make a difference. It is time for us to change the unhealthy interactions by changing our side of the relationship. Just as we can now use our imagery expertise to envision nursing as healthy and powerful, so can we create, first in our minds, the attitudes that will release us from unhealthy working relationships.

Allied Health Professionals

There are a great many types of allied health professionals. These people can also be enticed into the healing web through positive respect and healthy communications. All people involved in the care of the sick need to take excellent care of themselves and to learn to honor each of the various practitioners involved in caring for the patients we share. Teamwork and collaboration have a very healing effect on those involved, whether directly or peripherally.

The Family

Another way nurses can creatively inspire healthy relationships is to involve the patient's family in the promotion of healthy changes. Keep in mind that these people are also under enormous emotional pressure; it is valuable to teach the family members to channel the power of the mind in the healing of the family. Nurses are in a wonderful and unique position to effect positive change on the family unit.

Think about your patients and how much of their lives depend on the connections with their loved ones. Consider how much healthier the patients would be if they could be taught to communicate more clearly with family members.

Just as the nurse is able to learn to communicate with upset and hostile patients, so, too, can she begin to articulate how she might handle patients with their families. Most people are not well-trained in the art of assertiveness, yet nurses can be very sensitive to the energies spread by patients and family members.

We can be instrumental in inspiring changes without lecturing or being dogmatic or judgmental. By demonstrating how we have learned to talk to certain people in given situations, we become models for the families. Families can feel stronger in their abilities to care for the patients and still take care of themselves.

The Power of Assertive Communication

Consider the situation of Emily, a geriatric nurse in a large extended care facility. Emily has become very excited about the possibilities of using imagery in her work with clients. She has found that she can dramatically reduce the medications given on night shift for sleep if she takes the time to use gentle relaxation exercises with her agitated patients.

One evening, as she began to initiate a relaxation session with a particularly challenging patient, the patient's family dropped by, and Emily found them quite responsive to learning how to help the patient relax. She agreed to provide a relaxation session in their presence so they could learn to do the same.

Just as the patient became calm, the doctor stormed in to make quick rounds. Emily had already begun to help the patient breathe deeply, relax, and go to a special place when suddenly the door flew open and the doctor began to speak loudly. Emily motioned to the doctor to be quiet, and he became insulted. He began to shout about the lack of cooperation from nurses, and Emily found herself asking him to please step out in the corridor for a moment. She encouraged the patient to continue deep breathing and imagining how it felt to be in this special place.

Emily quietly slipped out into the hall and confronted the very upset physician. She allowed him to express his upset, then asked if he could hear her out. He agreed, and Emily explained what she had been doing, why she was doing it, and what the effects had been in recent times with this patient.

The doctor seemed perplexed, but he could see that she was quite adamant about this process. Emily then opened the patient's chart and demonstrated that the evenings when she had been able to use relaxation techniques were the times when the patient slept soundly and did not disturb others. Not only was the patient more cooperative, but he required much less medication, which eliminated many unpleasant side effects and costs.

The doctor seemed very interested after hearing all this, and was eager to witness the process. Emily invited him into the room and completed the short session with the patient. Afterward, the family asked a few simple questions and thanked Emily profusely. They seemed honored that the nurse would take this kind of time with them and their father, and they felt empowered to use these tools to help whenever they were around.

The end results were that the patient was much more cooperative on a regular basis, the family tended to take more time with their father and more interest in his care, and the doctor began to learn how to use relaxation techniques in his own practice with very positive results. In fact, it was the doctor who suggested that Emily create a sign that could be used by all staff on the unit. The sign was to say "Do not disturb for five minutes. Relaxation occurring—Relax!" There was good humor on the unit as staff and family bonded through the transmission of information about the use of gentle therapeutic imagery.

Nurses can convey to other health providers what has worked for them in special situations. In sharing our knowledge,

we inspire collaboration and teamwork. This type of enthusiasm and respect has far-reaching implications for the future of
health care.

HELPFUL HINTS

Keep in mind that imagery is a powerful tool for activating the
imagination. Our health care system today lacks opportunity for
enjoyment and humor. If we are to be effective in anything we
try, we need to allow for the involvement of creative imagination.

Special Precautions

There are certain clients who may not be appropriate for this type
of work. An example might be a client who has very low blood
pressure. Imagery might further lower the client's pressure to
encourage him to relax deeply.

Always be sure to get permission from the client. We can
never assume anything. We might wish for the client to be a certain way. It is much healthier, however, if we allow others to be
whoever they are. The client is always the best judge of whether
he is ready to face certain parts of himself and his life. It is our
responsibility to honor his decisions.

Another precaution is to know some of the background of
anyone you work with using imagery. Do a brief medical history.
Is the person anxious? Does he need a medihaler or nitroglycerin?
If so, be sure to have these essential items available prior to
entering into an imagery or relaxation experience. It is important
to have everything you might need in advance.

Also, find out about the client's medical and behavioral patterns. Does he have a psychiatric history? Has he ever given evidence of dissociative behavior? Is he connected to reality or is he
living in denial or fantasy? All of these considerations are important when attempting to ascertain appropriateness of techniques.

Another valuable piece of advice is this: Use the client's
words as much as possible. Do not use medical terminology,
which would instantly create a sense of discomfort, fear, or
shame. Pay attention to your client's use of words, and consider
it part of your creative challenge as a healer to be aligned with

his expression. Experience has taught the leaders in this type of work that the process is most effective when the guide speaks the same language as the client.

A final precaution at this point is a reminder: pay attention to your inner voice as you offer guidance. If you set aside some time to work with a client, but then discover that the person is particularly hungry at the moment, for example, it is not a good idea to insist on sticking to your plan. Similarly, if family is visiting the client, or the client would prefer time alone, the guide must be sensitive to the timing.

It is also important that the client is properly prepared. Should he need more information or documentation before embarking on this journey, his perceived needs should be considered foremost. In this way, we are building trust which will allow for a deeper healing in time.

Finally, as a precaution, be aware of how *you* are doing prior to working with anyone. If you are hungry, or tired, or upset, it may not be the best time to offer your services. When we deny our truth, we weaken our potential. When we, as healers, learn to be honest with ourselves and our process, we provide healthy role models and establish trust.

A Powerful Experience

A holistic physician had a very powerful experience using imagery. He was involved in an unusual healing program offered through a well-known holistic medical center. Because this clinic was considering hiring this doctor, he was asked to participate in its intensive healing program.

Part of the experience the program offered was three hours of massage to music. This process was specifically designed to relax the body completely and allow the mind to be creative while the spiritual essence was awakened and activated.

Midway through this experience, in a very somnambulistic state, the physician had a sensation of a hand on his heart. He was surprised, as he could feel the massage therapist's hands working on his feet. He looked up in his mind's eye, and saw an image of Jesus hovering over him, smiling down upon him and touching his heart. He was astounded.

He spoke to the image: "What are you doing here?" (This doctor was raised in the Jewish tradition and did not believe in Jesus as saviour.) Jesus smiled broadly, knowing instantly what he meant, and said, "No problem."

Before the doctor could say anything else, the image disappeared abruptly, and in its place, appeared Moses (much more familiar to the Hebrew doctor). This kind of "seeing" can be very healing and creative. In this instance, the vision helped the doctor to remember to honor the belief systems of the client. He was also reminded that the mind can be infinitely creative and flexible.

Creative Nursing

Nursing, as a profession, is changing rapidly. These ideas can provide a new lens for nurses, allowing us to be more willing to look at the same work in a new light. Nurses need to feel creative. We need to touch the people we work with on many levels.

In the Healing Touch Certification program, offered through the American Holistic Nurses Association (see Appendix), the touch component is added to healing work. This subtle energy work is a powerful complement to imagery sessions.

There are many ways in which nurses can be creative in their healing endeavors. The people we work with are unique and may respond differently to various interventions. Many nurses are using healing sound, movement, and art to access deeper levels of connection in the people with whom they work.

At times, patients will react in a strong manner to therapeutic maneuvers. We might even begin to witness some psychopathology that has not necessarily been evident in previous caring attempts. For this reason, nurses and patients might have some aversion to trying new tools. It is unlikely that anything unmanageable will occur, but because the images arise from the depth of the unconscious, it is valuable to have someone trained in psychotherapy available if there is any reason to be concerned about a patient's mental state. This may not be realistic in acute units, unless there is a psychiatric liaison nurse available, but it certainly is very practical in mental health units with adequate staffing. Working in this way, nurses can feel totally comfortable using creative methods to support the healing process of their patients.

Also keep in mind that something like this is very unlikely to occur in a brief experience. We have already ascertained that this type of tool is not used on someone who has displayed evidence of psychotic process.

Honoring Religious/Philosophical Orientations

It is helpful to keep in mind that there are certain religious groups that are uncomfortable with the aspect of emptying the mind. We must remember to pay attention to, and honor, people's beliefs.

As a brief example, I was living on a remote island years ago and was asked by a hospital to teach birthing classes. Many of the clientele were from other parts of the world, and though they spoke English, they exhibited a variety of culturally related health practices.

When I told the birthing class participants to empty their minds and take several deep breaths, a few of the participants walked out. Only later did I learn that these people were of a certain religious order, one that believed emptying the mind was the work of the devil!

We might begin by asking people if they have used any relaxation or breathing techniques. We can honor their fears by starting simply and noticing how open they are to progress.

If the clients are comfortable with prayer, we can support them in doing what makes sense and offers the most meaning to them. We can help to make the framework familiar and most comfortable.

Keep in mind that this kind of sensitivity is what differentiates between a nurse who uses her imagination and keeps her worklife creative and one who is more of a technician and practices rote tasks in a less interesting way.

We also need to keep in mind that there is no such thing as the "average nurse." All nurses come from different levels of belief and awareness.

Many academically oriented nurses have been working to bring the concepts of integrated care into the educational institutions. Slowly, steadily, there is an infiltration of nurses with new ways of thinking and working. Many other nurses, however, may not understand the process of viewing people as multidimensional beings. Change takes time and often needs to happen in a steady, progressive manner.

SUMMARY

Part of our new role as nurses will be to empower health care consumers, to enable them to make more and better decisions about their health choices. As we reach out, we will be seen as educators. We will also reach out to others to create a network of healing that will allow both patients and providers the healthiest possible conditions in which to grow and be nourished.

References

Carson, D., & Sams, J. (1988). *Medicine cards: The discovery of power through the ways of animals.* Santa Fe, NM: Bear & Company.

IMAGERY:
SEEING THE NURSE
AS HEALER

Physician: Heal Thyself

Socrates

A beautiful new book written by two nurses and a woman's healing expert offers a profound piece of wisdom for us to consider: "Many of us who work in the healing professions share a secret: When we act or work on another's behalf, we too are brought into harmonious relationship, we are made more whole." (Acterberg, Dossey, & Kolkmeier, 1994, p. 21)

In this simple wisdom, we become aware of one of the gifts of doing this work. As we align ourselves with our highest wisdom and our greatest internal resources, we have the most to share with those seeking our support. In helping others in this way, we help ourselves.

NURSING AS SACRED WORK

Using imagery for healing purposes is high-level nursing. This work, while simple, is also "sacred." The word, *sacred,* when used in this manner, refers to that which touches the soul. Nursing, when practiced with integrity, is sacred work. When we invite our clients to stretch themselves and reach into the deepest places of their souls, the work is sacred.

As guides and healers, we are asked to put ourselves aside and assist wholeheartedly in the growth of those entrusted to our care. To be able to do this and to do it well, we require special tools. It is not practical to suggest that we can enrich the lives of those we work with if we exist without joy, without sensitivity, without having faced our own darknesses.

THE WOUNDED HEALER ARCHETYPE

The myth of the Wounded Healer tells the story of Chiron, a centaur (half man, half horse). When Chiron visited a cave with other centaurs, they drank wine and lost control. A battle ensued in which Chiron was shot by an arrow. Chiron, though wounded, was able to offer instructions for the care of his wound. Because Chiron was immortal, he could not die. His wound, however, could not be cured, and thus he remained wounded. From that place of injury and knowledge, Chiron taught many healers how to care for others and to acknowledge their own woundedness.

Much of the literature about healing describes the healer as one who has faced both the dark and the light, who has seen the face of death and also the light of the eternal. The value of modern medicine has been lessened by a prevalent fear of acknowledging and facing the shadow side. The shadow side is that which is less pleasant and less socially acceptable. Our culture tends to ignore the gifts of the shadow, focusing instead on the peak experiences. Death, in the framework of modern medicine, has been the enemy.

In reality, however, death is a natural phenomenon, a necessary part of the life process. Most cultures from around the world seem to have created rituals that embrace all aspects of living and dying. Ours, on the other hand, has been death defying, with great heroic efforts dedicated to ignoring the positive aspects of this crucial life transition.

NURSING'S SPECIAL CHALLENGE

As hospital nurses who have chosen to identify strongly with the medical model adopt its death-defying stance, we may also have given up much of our power. Keep this in mind: *power* is the ability to influence change; *responsibility* is the ability to respond. We as nurses need to do both in our unique ways.

If we are to be identified as healers, we must be willing to consider the shadow and the light, the pain and the joy, the laughter and the tears, the birth and the death. To be responsible—that is, able to respond—we must come from our internal guidance in working with people and not accept blindly that which does not innately support our image as healers.

SECRETARY'S COMMISSION ON NURSING REPORT

In 1988, the United States government expressed its concern about the shortage of nurses by creating a committee to study the crisis. Many well-credentialed individuals from a variety of health-related professions worked together to examine and make recommendations about the nursing problem.

After a year of careful study, the Secretary's Commission on Nursing Report concluded the following:

> . . . the time has come to examine the role and functions of the nurse. The vital role of nursing in relation to American health care priorities must be articulated. A full and ongoing dialogue between nursing and its public is crucially important to the renegotiation of the contract between nursing and society. This is the essential task facing nursing and society over the next decade.

In this charge, nursing is being asked to clarify its vital role. It seems as if we have identified so strongly with medicine that we are in danger of losing all that is unique and relevant to our work. Nursing's soul has, in ancient times, been more closely related to the work of the ministry than that of the medical

profession. Yet we have been empowered with the task to articulate our unique role. Part of that role involves nurturing the
souls of our patients and providing physical care. Herein we can
make a distinction between "curing" and "caring."

CURING, CARING, AND HEALING

The following may help to clarify the uniqueness of nursing and
to understand the initial steps a nurse might take in incorporating imagery into her work. We first need to distinguish between
words that have been used somewhat interchangeably in the
world of medicine.

Curing often refers to the ability to remove symptoms. Many
nurses have seen patients leave the hospital asymptomatic, often
to return with similar, or different, symptoms later. Working
purely with symptoms is a crisis-oriented approach that does not
often produce profound or lasting results.

Caring, as we know, has often been considered to be the
unique domain of nursing. Realistically, however, caring is a
component that relates to all healing endeavors. Chiropractors,
physical therapists, doctors, and most other health professionals
claim caring as part of their domain. Nurses care in a unique way.

Healing, on the other hand, can involve components of
both curing and caring. From the Greek word *halos*, "to heal"
means to make whole. In healing work, the parts are synergisti-
cally blended to weave a beautiful tapestry that allows all aspects
of one's being to blend into a unique presentation. Nursing work,
when it is healing, honors the many parts of a person and
inspires an acceptance and respect for the whole.

In understanding the difference between these terms, we
can arrive at a special appreciation for the challenge of nursing
as it moves into the twenty-first century.

HEALING RITUALS

In their book *Rituals of Healing*, Acterberg, Dossey, and
Kolkmeier (1994) make a number of suggestions to support peo-

ple on their healing journeys. The authors encourage the seeker to consider illness a rite of passage. This is a powerful thought. It inspires us to eliminate the judgments we hold about illness and disease.

Further, it asks us to consider viewing illness as a challenge to be met with sacred intent, rather than as a punishment for some vague or specific transgression. The gift of this approach is the reminder that each of us can always decide how to face any of life's challenges, and can view these times of transition as growth opportunities.

The authors suggest three phases to the process: the separation phase, the transition phase, and the return. These aspects are reflected from the myth of the hero's journey, when a seeker leaves to face darkness and returns enlightened.

The Hero's Journey: Initial Phase

In the initial phase of this journey, Acterberg, Dossey, and Kolkmeier acknowledge that crisis is often the precipitating inspiration for change. When facing a crisis, we often must face a change of scene. It is further suggested that there are ways to augment or simulate this change.

Several suggestions for facing this experience include finding a healing space (the authors suggest that one choose to view the hospital as a healing place); feeling a sense of connectedness to ancestors, blood relatives, or chosen family; purifying the environment in such a way as to make it feel sacred; and enacting some sort of ritualistic break with the old. This can be done within a group setting to empower the process and is most effective when it arises from the psyche of the person undergoing transition.

The Hero's Journey: Transition Phase

In this phase, the seeker faces both darkness and light in efforts to learn more about his own true nature. It is considered to be a time between worlds, when the old way of being has ended but the new one has not yet fully begun. It is a journey into the void, the unknown, where one must face one's fears and seek the path to one's personal growth.

The authors of *Rituals of Healing* suggest several actions to be undertaken during this time of transition. The first of these is taking time alone. Illness is certainly an opportunity to take time alone, and people facing illness often feel isolated.

To cope with this aspect, it is suggested that the person consider that he is experiencing a symbolic death and rebirth. Seeing transition in this light helps us all to think in terms larger than the moment; to see our experiences and those of our patients as opportunities to reconnect to a spiritual source, which gives us sustenance and courage.

Along with this idea comes the notion that while undergoing this journey, there is extraordinary help available. Friends gather around, and the artistic expressions of life's poignancy help us to reframe our experience. Acterberg, Dossey, and Kolkmeier suggest that relaxation and imagery play important roles in changing consciousness to promote recovery. We see and feel things differently. Our dreams may become more significant at this time.

Then, we might further empower our process with some positive rehearsal, in which we anticipate the future and plan for it in a positive light. We might also seek the wisdom of others who have traveled this path before us. This transition phase is a time of gathering.

The Hero's Journey: Return Phase

In this final phase, the seeker returns to where he once lived. The surroundings might be the same, but the seeker has changed, and thus he responds differently. There may be new challenges to face, and the seeker must remember to take care of himself in the midst of the ordinary and extraordinary demands.

It is often beneficial to initiate some sort of break with the past and to commit to the new life. Feelings must be transformed before the person is free to move on.

All of this preparation is what is asked of our patients when we serve as their nurses in their times of need. More important to remember, however, is that to support our patients in the recovery of their sense of wholeness, we nurses likewise must face our own journeys.

THE NURSE'S JOURNEY

We have already explored the idea of nursing as sacred work. We have considered the "hero's journey," in which the seeker travels to learn about the self. We have examined the importance of becoming role models to inspire health in others. Now we will contemplate some initial steps for nurses on the healing journey.

Become Your Own Hero

One of the first steps, then, might be to consider that just as our patients are travelers on the road to recovery and healing, so are we travelers on that same road. Much that we were taught in our nursing school curricula focused on external manipulations. By beginning to see ourselves as healers, we can release any fear or arrogance and allow ourselves to be extremely vulnerable, and possibly naive.

Most nurses have not considered what is truly required of those doing healing work. We have been indoctrinated into a culture that worships science and technology, and we may have forgotten to honor the power of belief, rituals, and prayer. When we return to our roots, honoring that which is ancient and universal, and attempt to incorporate some healing modalities, we must be willing to embark on our own journeys into wholeness. For a scientific explanation we may look to current research.

Bandura's Studies

A Stanford University psychologist has spent many years doing research on empowerment issues. Dr. Albert Bandura (1990) has published a number of papers in respected scientific journals related to the concept of empowerment. In these studies, Dr. Bandura and his fellow researchers have found that one of the key components in empowerment is what he calls *mastery modeling*. In mastery modeling, the expert is able to convey knowledge through behavior. This concept allows for empowerment through sharing skills, tools, information, and support, all of which can be utilized to promote healthy, beneficial change.

What Dr. Bandura has been able to prove scientifically is something many of us have known intuitively; that we learn more from observing the actions of others than we do from merely listening to what we are told. In other words, the old adage "Do what I say, not what I do" is not what happens in real life. We are most apt to learn from the modeling behavior of others.

Mastery modeling refers to modeling that one has mastered. In being fully who one is and acting from one's source of power, others benefit. To put it simply, actions speak louder than words.

Nursing Modeling Theory

Another theorist, this time from within the ranks of the nursing profession, has based her nursing theories on concepts she calls *modeling* and *role modeling*. Helen Erickson (1983) has recently excited the imagination of nursing theorists and students alike with her ideas about modeling and role modeling. There are academic conferences taking place around the country that are devoted to exploring Erickson's ideas as they relate to nursing practice. This work allows the nurse to "walk in the patient's moccasins," and attempt to feel like the patient might in his situation. All of this creative work involves imagery—using the power of the mind to create healthy change.

Thus, we can begin to see the importance of representing that which we wish to portray. To begin to offer healing modalities, we may wish to align our image with that of someone who represents health. The beauty of this process is that as we learn the natural healing tools, we simultaneously learn to heal ourselves. The gift is twofold: we enhance our own well-being while becoming models of health for those entrusted to our care.

Imagine Yourself a Healer

(**Note:** *You might read this initially, then come back later to experience it. You can also read it slowly into a tape player, then play the tape back so you can relax and practice your own visualizations.)*

We will now do an imagery experience to use our minds to change our minds. If you have not viewed yourself as a healer, this is an opportunity to begin to see yourself and your work differently. If you have seen yourself as a healer, this is your opportunity to strengthen your vision.

At this time, I invite you to find a relaxing place where you can be quiet and contemplative for a while. You might want to put signs on the door, unplug the phone, and do all the things you might also do if you were providing an imagery session for a client. This time, however, you are your client.

Sit comfortably, and become aware of your feet as they touch the floor. Close your eyes, and take several slow, deep breaths. Breathe in fully and deeply through the nose, blowing out fully and strongly through the mouth. Continue to inhale and exhale slowly, feeling yourself being revitalized by the breath.

Feel your feet on the floor. As you breathe in fully, allow your mind to focus on the soles of your feet. Imagine that you can see holes in the center of the sole of each foot. From this hole, picture a strong root growing from inside your being, coming out through this foot opening, and burrowing to the center of the earth. Feel your connection with the earth. Allow yourself to feel well-planted on the earth, supported by the earth's wisdom and energy.

As you breathe, you breathe in Earth energy and wisdom. As you breathe, you breathe out anything that no longer serves your highest good. Breathe in strength, beauty, and wisdom; blow out sadness, pain, negativity. Breathe in love, blow out fear; breathe in courage, blow out anything that feels heavy or dense in your being. Use this as a time to recharge, a time to allow the body to release anything that has been stored during times of stress or pain.

Be sure to appreciate your body at this time of healing. Thank it for all it does to keep you functioning and pain-free. If you have pain, be aware of that discomfort and honor it for the message it brings.

This is a time to create a new relationship with your body. This is a time to create a new relationship with your mind. This is a time to acknowledge the gifts you have, the strengths you have developed, and the many blessings in your life. It can also be a time to make a commitment to yourself.

You might tell yourself: 'From this moment on, I choose to be happy. From this moment on, I agree to listen to my body and to pay attention to its subtle signals. I am now committed to healing myself so I can help others to heal. I am an instrument for healing, and I am committed to healing my body so I can be of service to others in my life.'

This is a time of transformation. This is a time of planetary healing; this is a time for major changes. Every one of us has a role in the new paradigm, and we need to stay healthy to model leadership for others.

This is a new age for nursing. Never before have we had such an opportunity to impact change. Never before have nurses been in a position to impact the welfare of nations as we are today. Never before have we had the media and technology to advance our cause so radically.

As you continue to relax and breathe deeply, imagine yourself in your highest vision of your life. Imagine yourself doing exactly what you love to do, doing it well, and receiving acknowledgment and recognition for your contributions. Imagine that you wake up each morning delighted to be who you are and thrilled to be able to do your work and to have such incredible support for your dreams.

Imagine that you are surrounded by others who have agreed to be part of your mastermind team, people who are committed to the healing of the planet in the same ways that you are. Imagine that all these people support your deepest heart's desire and wish only the best for you. Imagine being surrounded by the kind of love that every child wishes and dreams of, and though now it may be coming from people who may or may not be your blood relatives, they are related through the passion you share. They are your chosen family, and you feel rich and blessed.

Now imagine yourself as a healer. Picture that you feel connected to your source, and strong. You feel aligned with your highest abilities, and you know that you are guided in your work. You feel your connection to your highest self and to others, and you also feel very connected to life. You feel certain of your abilities, proud of your accomplishments, eager to make your special contributions, and proud to be a nurse.

You have gained a sense of mastery over your own well-being, and you are committed to helping others accomplish that for themselves. You are a teacher, showing the way to personal power and joy. You are a guide, introducing some of life's most healing opportunities to all you work with, and you exude a sense of strength and compassion.

You have learned from all of your experiences. You have accepted the pain and the loss with the beauty and the success. You feel balanced in the way you live, and find yourself surrounded by people who love and support you.

You have become clear and strong. You have learned your life lessons well, and now you are amongst the chosen for providing a new model of power. You are living proof that one can be strong, yet gentle, effective, and joyful.

You love to use your hands in your healing work. You feel it is part of your mission to touch people in your special way, to make a difference in their lives, to support their healthy endeavors. You find that your heart and head are aligned, and that you feel at peace as you move through the world, showering those you contact with a sense of peace and love.

You are a healer. You help others to feel whole and holy. You feel connected to your Higher Power at all times, and you inspire others to reconnect with their source of love and strength, whatever they consider that source to be. You have learned to set healthy boundaries, to honor people for their special contributions, and to support each person's growth and empowerment. You are a healer.

Now, picture yourself surrounded by other nurses who are also healers. These nurses feel great about their work, they love what they do, and they are a joy to work with.

These nurses are also committed to being part of the change. They are no longer content to witness maltreatment, either of clients or nurses, and together you are bonded in an ancient and communal way. You feel good knowing these other nurses, you have learned to trust yourself and to trust them, and you have learned to join forces for the creation of a most powerful healing team. All of you feel whole and centered in your lives and work, and when you join forces, there is an unmistakable synergy that allows for tremendous healing to occur.

You have learned to work together for the betterment of your lives. You have learned to work together for the enhancement of your health care facilities. You have learned to work together for the healing of the planet.

Through your endeavors, the world is experiencing major healing. Nurses are now active in the communities, bringing back the nurturing touch, the loving care, and a new model for strength.

Nurses are in leadership positions across the world, teaching people about healthy options. We are using our vast creativity to build a healthier world, one that supports all people regardless of race, creed, or nation.

It is a joy to be a nurse today. It feels wonderful to know that you are making a difference. It is thrilling to be on the cutting edge, to represent the feminine principle in health care. We are delighted with our many, diverse roles.

Nurses are reaching out to people in need with loving arms and healing hearts. We are Health Educators, Life Transition Guides, models of gentle power. We touch our patients deeply, in ways that inspire the will to be well.

Imagine that nursing is now considered a time-honored profession. Your colleagues are mutually supportive, happy, and healthy. We have learned so much, and we are now in a position to share our knowledge with compassion and humor.

Imagine that all these healthy changes were implemented because each nurse assumed the responsibility for working on her little piece of the puzzle. Each nurse learned to heal herself and to imagine, and so it was that nursing became a most powerful profession.

Imagine that you were a part of the transformation. As you made decisions about how your life needed to be and found within yourself the courage to bring those visions to reality, you felt better and better about your life, and you inspired others to feel better about theirs.

SUMMARY

As nurses become creative, as we begin to accept and acknowledge who we are and what our special gifts are, we become leaders in the health care industry. Use your mind to imagine nursing powerful, imagine nurses feeling whole, and healthy, and modeling these aspects of wholeness for their clients.

The mind is our most valuable tool. Nurse-healers are changing their minds about nursing and preparing to change the world of health care. You can help in this endeavor. Change your mind and you change the world.

References

Acterberg, J., Dossey, B., & Kolkmeier, L. (1994). *Rituals of healing.* New York: Bantam.

Bandura, A. (1990). Mechanisms governing empowerment effects: A self-efficacy analysis. *Journal of Personality & Social Psychology, 58,* 472–486.

Department of Health & Human Services. (1988). *Secretary's commission on nursing. Final Report, Vol. I.* Washington, DC: U.S. Government Printing Office.

RESOURCE GUIDE

In addition to the references listed at the end of each chapter, the author refers the reader to the following resources for additional related information.

Books and Articles

Achterberg, J. (1985). *Imagery in healing; Shamanism and modern medicine.* Boston: New Science Library.

Achterberg, J., & Lawlis, F. (1980). *Bridges of the bodymind: Behavioral approaches to health care.* Champaign, IL: Institute for Personality and Behavior Testing.

Achterberg, J., Dossey, B., Kolkmeier, L. (1994). *Rituals of healing: Using imagery for health and wellness.* New York: Bantam. (Has excellent extensive bibliography)

Anderson, G. (1988). *The cancer conquerer.* Kansas City, KS: Andrews and McMeel.

Assagioli, R. (1965). *Psychosynthesis: A manual of principles and techniques.* New York: Hobbs, Doorman and Co.

Barbach, L. (1975). *For yourself: The fulfillment of female sexuality.* New York: Doubleday & Co.

Barbach, L., & Levine, L. (1980). *Shared intimacies.* New York: Doubleday & Co.

Barber, T.X. (1974). *Hypnosis, imagination and human potentialities.* New York: Pergamon Press.

Barlow, W. (1973). *The Alexander technique.* New York: Alfred A. Knopf.

Benson, H. (1975). *Beyond relaxation response.* New York: Avon Books.

Benson, H. (1975). *Relaxation response.* New York: Avon Books.

Bertherat, T., & Bernstein, C. (1977). *The body has its reasons: Anti-exercises and self-awareness.* New York: Pantheon Books.

Borysenko, J. (1979). *Minding the body, mending the mind.* Menlo Park, CA: Addison-Wesley.

Bresler, D., & Trubo, R. (1979). *Free yourself from pain.* New York: Simon & Shuster.

Bry, A. *Visualization: Directing the movies of your mind.* New York: Barnes & Noble.

Chopra, D. (1989). *Quantam healing.* New York: Bantam Books.

Crampton, M. (1977). *A historical survey of mental imagery techniques in psychotherapy and description of the dialogic imaginal method.* Montreal, Quebec: Quebec Center for Psychosynthesis, Inc.

Dossey, B., Keenan, L., Guzzetta, C., & Kolkmeier, L. (1995). *Holistic nursing: A handbook for practice.* (2nd ed.). Gaithersberg, MD: Aspen Publishers.

Dossey, L. (1989). *Recovering the soul.* New York: Bantam Books.

Dossey, L. (1993). *Healing words: The power of prayer and the practice of medicine.* San Francisco: HarperCollins.

Ellis, J., Isaac, W., & Isaac, D. (1989). *The wellness therapy handbook: Using relaxation and visualization for the management of hemophilia and HIV.* Winnipeg, Manitoba, Canada: Canadian Hemophilia Society, Wellness Therapy Project.

Erickson, H., Tomlin, E., & Swain, M. (1983). *Modelling and role modelling: A theory and paradigm for nursing.* Lexington, SC: Pine Press.

Ferrucci, P. (1982). *What we may be: Techniques for psychological growth.* Los Angeles: J.P. Tarcher, Inc.

Gawain, S. (1983). *Creative visualization.* Berkeley, CA: Whatever Publishing.

Gendlin, E. (1981). *Focusing.* New York: Bantam Books.

Green, E., & Green, A. (1977). *Beyond biofeedback.* New York: Delacorte Press.

Hall, H. (1982, October). Hypnosis and the immune system: A review with implications for cancer and the psychology of healing. *American Journal of Clinical Hypnosis.* October–January, Vol. 25, #2–3, pp. 92–103.

Halprin, A. (1979). *Movement ritual.* San Francisco: San Francisco Dancers' Workshop.

Halprin, A., & Nixon, J.H. (1977). *Dance as a self healing art.* San Francisco: San Francisco Dancers' Workshop.

Hilgard, E.R., & Hilgard, J. (1983). *Hypnosis in the relief of pain.* Los Altos, CA: William Kaufmann, Inc.

Horowitz, M. (1970). *Image formation and cognition.* New York: Meredith Corp.

Hutschnecker, A. (1953). *The will to live.* London, England: Thomas Y. Crowell.

Jaffe, D.T. (1979). *Healing from within.* New York: Knopf.

Jampolsky, G. (1975). *A course in miracles.* Tiburon, CA: Foundation for Inner Peace.

Jampolsky, G. (1979). *Love is letting go of fear.* Millbrae, CA: Celestial Arts.

Jaynes, J. (1983). *The consequences of consciousness.* New York: Houghton Mifflin.

Johnson, R. (1986). *Inner work.* San Francisco: Harper and Row.

Kenner, C. (1985). Burn injury. In C. Kenner, C. E. Guzzetta, & B. M. Dossey (Eds.), *Critical care nursing: Body-mind-spirit* (pp. 1135–1137). Boston, MA: Little, Brown and Co.

Kenner, C. (1985). Extremity trauma. In C. Kenner, C. E. Guzzetta, & B. M. Dossey (Eds.), *Critical care nursing: Body-mind-spirit.* Boston, MA: Little, Brown and Co.

Knowles, R. (1984). *A guide to self-management strategies for nurses.* New York: Springer Publishing Co.

Korn, E., & Johnson, K. (1983). *Visualization: The uses of imagery in the health professions.* Homewood, IL: Dow Jones-Irwin.

Kroger, W.S., & Fegler, W. D. (1976). *Hypnosis & behavior modification: Imagery conditioning.* Philadelphia: J.B. Lippincott.

Lazarus, A. (1977). *In the mind's eye: The power of imagery for personal enrichment.* New York: Guilford Press.

LeShan, L. (1974). *How to meditate.* New York: Bantam Books.

LeShan, L. (1989). *Cancer as a turning point.* New York: E.P. Dutton & Co.

Ley, R.G. (1979). Cerebral asymmetries, emotional experience, and imagery: Implications for psychotherapeutic change. In A.A. Sheikh & J. Shaffer (Eds.), *The potential of fantasy and imagination.* New York: Brandon House.

Locke, S. (1986). *The healer within.* New York: New American Library.

Lynch, J. (1985). *The language of the heart.* New York: Basic Books.

Mason, L. J. (1980). *Guide to stress reduction.* Culver City, CA: Peace Press.

McKim, R.H. (1972). *Experiences in visual thinking.* Monterey, CA: Brooks–Cole.

Morris, F. (1975). *Self hypnosis in two days.* New York: E. P. Dutton & Co.

Ornish, D. (1977). *The psychology of consciousness.* New York: Harcourt, Brace, Janovich, Inc.

Oyle, I. (1974). *The healing mind.* Millbrae, CA: Celestial Arts.

Oyle, I., & Jean, S. (1993). *The wizdom within.* Tiburon, CA: HJ Kramer, Inc.

Pelletier, K.R. (1978). *Holistic medicine from stress to optimum health.* New York: Delcorte Press-Seymour Lawrence.

Pelletier, K.R. (1979). *Mind as healer, mind as slayer.* New York: Delcorte Press-Seymour Lawrence.

Porter, G., & Norris, P. (1985). *Why me: Harnessing the healing power of the human spirit.* Walpole, NH: Stillpoint Publishers.

Pribram, K. (1982). *Languages of the brain.* (5th ed.). New York: Brandon House. (1st edition published 1971 by Prentice-Hall.)

Pribram, K., & Broadbent, D. (Eds.). (1970). *Biology of memory.* New York: Academic Press.

Progoff, I. (1963). *The symbolic and the real.* New York: Julian Press.

Rancour, P. (1991). "Guided Imagery: Healing When Curing is Out of the Question" in *Perspectives in Psychiatric Care.* Vol. 27, #4, pp. 30–33.

Remen, N. (1980). *The human patient.* Garden City, NY: Doubleday/Anchor Books.

Richardson, A. (1969). *Mental imagery.* New York: Springer Publishing Co.

Rivlin, R., & Gravelle, K. (1984). *Deciphering the senses: The expanding world of human perception.* New York: Simon & Schuster.

Rossi, E.L. (1986). *The psychobiology of mind-body healing: New concepts of therapeutic hypnosis.* New York: W.W. Norton.

Rossman, M. (1987). *Healing yourself: A step-by-step program to better health through imagery.* New York: Walker & Co.

Rossman, M., & Remen, N. (1981). *Imagine health! Imagery and insight in self-care.* Mill Valley, CA: Insight Publishing.

Samuels, M., & Samuels, N. (1975). *Seeing with the mind's eye: The history, techniques and uses of visualization.* New York: Random House.

Shaffer, M. (1982). *Life after stress.* New York: Plenum Press.

Shames, R., & Sterin, C. (1978). *Healing with mind power.* Emmaus, PA: Rodale Press.

Sheikh, A. (Ed.). (1982). *Imagery: Current theory, research and application.* New York: Wiley & Sons.

Sheikh, A. (Ed.). (1986). *Anthology of imagery techniques.* Milwaukee, WI: American Imagery Institute.

Shorr, J.E. (1977). *Go see the movie in your head.* New York: Popular Library.

Siegel, B. (1986). *Love, medicine, and miracles.* New York: Harper & Row.

Simonton, C., & Matthews-Simonton, S. (1978). *Getting well again.* Los Angeles: J.P. Tarcher, Inc.

Singer, J.L. (1974). *Imagery and daydream methods in psychotherapy.* New York: Academic Press.

Singer, J.L. (1975). *The inner world of daydreaming.* New York: Harper & Row.

Singer, J.L., & Pope, K. (1978). *The power of human imagination.* New York: Plenum.

Sommer, R. (1978). *The mind's eye.* New York: Delta.

Starker, S. (1982). *Fantastic thoughts: Dreams, daydreams, hallucinations and hypnosis.* Englewood Cliffs, NJ: Prentice-Hall.

Tart, C. (1975). *States of consciousness.* New York: E.P. Dutton.

Watkins, M. (1984). *Waking dreams.* Dallas: Spring Publications.

Tapes

Bresler, D. *Relaxation/Guided imagery & lecture tapes.* Los Angeles, CA: LA Healing Arts Center.

Davenport, L. *"Well spring" relaxation & imagery tape.* San Rafael, CA.

Dossey, B., & Keegan, L. (1987) *Self-care: A program to improve your life.* Temple, TX: BodyMind Systems.

Ezra, S. *Relaxation/Guided imagery tapes & instruction.* San Rafael, CA.

Fryling, V. *Autogenic training and visualization.* Oakland, CA: Audio Education Cassettes.

Miller, E. *Extensive catalog of imagery tapes.* Stanford, CA: Source Cassettes.

Mosher, M. *Inner peace* ("Flight to Freedom" tape with guided imagery and music). Angwin, CA: Health Education Resources.

Rossman, M. *Set of 6 instructional tapes of healing imagery.* Mill Valley, CA.

Siegel, B. *Guided imagery exercises and lecture tapes.* New Haven, CT: ECaP.

Simonton, O.C. *Tapes using imagery for cancer patients.* Pacific Palisades, CA.

Associations, Organizations and Programs

Academy for Guided Imagery, P.O. Box 2070, Mill Valley, CA 94942

American Holistic Nurses Association, 4101 Lake Boone Trail, Suite 201, Raleigh, NC 27607

"Beyond Ordinary Nursing" Workshops, 700 E Street, Suite 220, San Rafael, CA 94901; 415-453-6208.

Bridging the World, P.O. Box 1866, Soquel, CA 95073.

Cancer Support & Education Center, 1035 Pine St., Menlo Park, CA 94025

Certificate Program in Holistic Nursing, 24 South Prospect St., Amherst, MA 01002

Colorado Center for Healing Touch, 198 Union Blvd., Suite 210, Lakewood, CO 80228

Commonweal (alternative cancer treatment using imagery and other healing practices), P.O. Box 316, Bolinas, CA 94924

You can also locate the American Society of Clinical Hypnosis, Society for Clinical and Experimental Hypnosis, and the Academy of Hypnosis and American Psychological Society (Division of Psychological Hypnosis) in major cities across the United States.

To be placed on a mailing list for "Healing Journeys," conferences, etc., call 1-800-423-9882.

I N D E X

A

Academy for Guided Imagery, 54, 63
Addiction, imagery and, 102–105
Addictive thinking, imagery and, 103–104
Affirmation
  defined, 101
  imagery and, 101–102
Age progressions, 128–129
Alcoholism, imagery and, 105
Allergies, autoimmune imagery and, 137
American Holistic Nurses Association, Healing
    Touch Certification, 140
American Medical Association, hypnosis and, 43
Anger, health and, 138–139
Animal magnetism, theory of, 41
Antepartum imagery, 99–100
Antibiotics, imagery and, 81–82
Anxiety, dealing with, 83–84
Archetypes, Carl Jung and, 45
A.R.E. (Association for Research and Enlightenment),
    11
Aristotle
  emotion and, 40
  mind–body connection and, 65
Assertive communication, 194–195
Association for Research and Enlightenment
    (A.R.E.), 11
Athletes, image reversal and, 108
Audio tapes, for patients, 83
Autoimmune imagery, 137–138
Awareness, self, barriers to, 7–8

B

Bandura, Albert, studies by, 207–208
Benson, Herbert, relaxation response and, 64–65

Bernheim, Hippolyte, hypnosis and, 43
"Beyond Ordinary Nursing" imagery workshop,
    150
Birth–related imagery, 100–101, 108–109
Bodies
  feedback to, 5
  pain, as a messenger to, 5–6
Body–mind nursing, 149–150
Breathing
  childbirth and, 108–109
  counting, 84
  deepening relaxation response and, 76–77
  working with, 83
Bresler, David, Academy for Guided Imagery
    and, 54, 63
British Medical Society, hypnosis and, 43

C

California Nurses Association, on relaxation, 98
Cancer pain, imaging, 109
Caring, described, 204
Cartesian dualism, hypnosis and, 42
Cayce, Edgar, 11
The Center for Attitudinal Healing, 18
Changing–the–mind channel, 175–176
Childbirth pain, breathing and, 108–109
Chopra, Deepok, 10
Chronic pain. See Pain
Clients
  emotional experiences, guiding clients through,
    92
  resources of, utilizing, 150
Clinical practice
  dialogue with symptoms and, 112, 114–115
  inner guide

accessing, 91–92
guidelines for, 88–89
introducing, 88
meeting, 87–93
intermediate imagery, 93–99
legal considerations, 97–98
pain imagery techniques, 108–111
intensity scale and, 111–112
suggestions for, 93
See also Nurses
Codependency, 125–126
issues concerning, 171–172
Communication
assertive, 194–195
choices in, 183–185
Consciousness, Carl Jung and, 45–46
Countdown technique, 74–75
Creative
nursing, 198–199
visualization, 53–54, 71
Creative imaging
changing–the–mind channel, 175–176
decisional affirmation, 178–179
visual affirmation, 176–177
Creative Visualization, 53
Cultural images, Carl Jung on, 47
Curing, described, 204

D
Death
culture and, 202
imagery and, 136–137
Decisional affirmation, 178–179
Deepening relaxation response, 76–77
Descartes, René, 66
Cartesian dualism and, 42
mind–body connection and, 65
Diabetes, autoimmune imagery and, 137
Dialogue with symptoms, 112, 114–115
Disease, defined, 8
Doctors
introducing imagery to, 188–189
relationships with nurses, 193
Dreams, symbolic value of, 44–45

E
Educators, health, nurses as, 9–10
Emotional experiences, guiding clients through, 92
Emotions
Aristotle's view of, 40
Carl Jung on, 48
defined, 17

healing power of, 17–19
Empowerment: The Art of Creating Your Life As You Want It, 62
Empowerment, described, 61–62
Energetic research, energy flows and, 131
Energy flows, energetic research and, 131
Erickson, Helen, on role modeling, 208
Estes, Clarissa Pinkola, 50–52
Eternal truths, 47
Etheric body, healing of, 140–141
Eye muscle tightening and relaxing technique, 75
Ezra, Susan
imaging pain and, 110
interview with, 146–150
thoughts from, 150–153
work of, 83–84

F
False memory syndrome, 126–127
Fear
dealing with, 83–84
of the unknown, 48–49
working with, 84
Feedback, pain as, 5
Feeling, Jung's definition of, 45
Free Yourself from Pain, 54
Freud, Sigmund, hypnosis and, 43

G
Glove anesthesia technique, 110–111
Greeks, use of hypnosis by, 39–41
Guidance, contacting, 132–133
Guide
described, 72
See also Inner advisor
Guided imagery, 33, 53–54, 71
introductory session, 21–31
analysis of, 32
concepts concerning, 34–36

H
Habits
imagery and, 102–104
unhealthy, imagery and, 104–105
Harvey, William, Cartesian dualism and, 42
Hashimoto's disease, autoimmune imagery and, 137
Healer
imaging self as, 208–213
nurse as, 62–63
Healing
circle, 130
defined, 7

described, 204
emotions, power of, 17–19
of etheric body, 140–141
guidance to, 6–9
Lisa's adventure in, 156–159
loss, with imagery, 132–133
Middle Ages and, 66
nurse's journey of, 207–208
rituals, 204–206
teams, creating, 133–134
weaving the web of, 187–196
Healing Touch Certification, 140
Healing with Mind Power, 53
Healing Yourself: A Step-by-Step Program for Better Health Through Imagery, 54
Health
  anger and, 138–139
  planting images and, 126–127
Health educator, nurses as, 9–10
Higher sense perception, 131–132
Hill, Napoleon, 10
  Think & Grow Rich, 15
Hirshberg, Caryle, 165
  on long–term survival, 166
Hypnosis
  Cartesian dualism and, 42
  defined, 38, 72
  describe, 38–39
  eighteenth/nineteenth centuries and, 42–43
  imagery compared to, 38
  twentieth century and, 43
  use of, 39
    ancient Greeks, 39–41
    Middle Ages, 41
    Renaissance, 41–42

I

Image
  Carl Jung on, 48
    cultural, 47
  defined, 11, 70
  planting, 126–127
  power of, 11–15
  reversal, 108
  sources/effect of, 13–15
  terminology of, 64–66
    evolution of, 66–73
Imagery
  addictions and, 102–104
  addictive thinking and, 103–104
  affirmations and, 101–102
  alcoholism and, 105
  autoimmune, 137–138

beginning nurses and, 94–95
birth–related
  antepartum, 99–100
  labor, 100
  postpartum, 100–101
Carl Jung's contributions to, 43–49
clinical uses of, 63–64
death and, 136–137
defined, 32–33, 70
guided, 53–54, 71
  defined, 33
habits and, 102–104
  unhealthy and, 104–105
healing loss through, 132–133
hypnosis compared to, 38
interactive guided, 34
  defined, 72
intermediate, 93–99
intravenous fluids and, 81
introduction to
  of doctors, 188–189
  of patients, 189–190
making time for, 95–96
  examples of, 96–97
miscellaneous uses of, 99
nurse's role in, 59–64
oncology and, 106–108
procedure, 73–75
Scientific Revolution and, 66
spiritual uses of, 139–140
techniques for pain
  breathing, 108–109
  glove anesthesia, 110–111
  imaging pain and, 109–110
therapeutic, defined, 33, 71
Imagery session
  introductory, 21–31
    analysis of, 32
    concepts concerning, 34–36
Influence, avoiding negative, 135–136
Initiation rituals, Carl Jung on, 49
Inner advisor
  accessing, 91–92, 181–182
  body tour, deepening technique and, 77
  child, healing the, 125–126
  described, 72–73
  guidelines for, 88–89
  introducing, 88
  meeting, 87–93
  regression with, 124–125
Inner sensations, deepening technique and, 77
Instincts, Carl Jung and, 45
Institute of Noetic Science, 165

Intensity scale, pain and, 111–112
Interactive Guided Imagery, 34
  defined, 72
Interviews
  Jan Maxwell, 146–150
  Karilee Halo Shames, 146–150
  Susan Ezra, 146–150
Intravenous fluids, imagery and, 81
Introductory experience, 21–31
  analysis of, 32
  concepts concerning, 34–36
Intuition
  defined, 15
  Jung's definition of, 45
  use of, 15–17
IVs, imagery and, 81

J
Jampolsky, Gerald, 10, 138
  The Center for Attitudinal Healing and, 18
Jung, Carl
  on archetypes, 45
  on consciousness, 45–46
  contribution of, 43–49
  on cultural images, 47
  on dreams, 44–45
  on emotions, 48
  on the fear of the unknown, 48–49
  on images, 48
  impact of, 49–50
  on initiation ritual, 49
  on instinct, 45
  Man and His Symbols, 44
  on mythology, 46–47
  on psyche, 46
  on reason, 48
  on symbology, 46–47, 49

K
Keck, Anna, on self–healing, 163–167

L
Labor imagery, 100
Law, clinical practice and, 97–98
Life
  enhancing quality of, 174–175
  regressions, 130–131
  transitions, working with, 122
Loss, confronting, 115

M
Mandino, Og, 10

Man and His Symbols, 44
Man's Search for Meaning, 12
Mastery modeling, described, 207–208
Matthews–Simonton, Stephanie, 12, 71
  oncology imagery and, 106–107
  research by, 69
Maxwell, Jan
  interview with, 146–150
  thoughts from, 153–156, 159–160
Mesmer, Franz, theory of animal magnetism and,
    41
Middle Ages
  healing and, 66
  use of hypnosis during, 41
Miller, Terry
  on imagery, 168–170
  imagery in nursing and, 81
Mind, power of, 10–11
Mind As Healer, Mind As Slayer, 10
Mind–body connection, 65
Mythology, Carl Jung on, 46–47

N
Nacebo effect, described, 10–11
National Institutes of Health, Candace Pert and,
    68–69
Natural symbols, described, 47
Negative influence, avoiding, 135–136
Neuropeptides, immunity and, 68
Newman, Margaret, on pattern recognition, 114
Nightingale, Florence, on healing, 59–60
Nurse Practice Act, 98
Nurses
  as healers, 62–63
  as health educators, 9–10
  imagery and, 59–64, 94–95
  journey of healing, 207–208
  patient's family and, 193–194
  relationships with doctors, 193
  See also Clinical practice
Nursing
  body–mind, 149–150
  care, whole body, 179–181, 183
  challenge of, 203
  creative, 198–199
  as sacred work, 201–202

O
Oncology, imagery in, 106–108
Open–mindedness, developing, 96
Osler, Sir William, mind–body connection and,
    65

P

Pain
  as a body messenger, 5–6
  breathing and, 108–109
  dynamics of chronic, 4–5
  glove anesthesia technique, 110–111
  image of, 109–110
  intensity scale and, 111–112
  medications, imagery and, 81
  metaphors of, 114–115
  sacred space creation and, 118–119
Pasteur, Louis, germ theory and, 43
Past life regressions, 130–131
Patients
  introducing imagery to, 189–190
  tapes for, 83
Pelletier, Kenneth, *Mind As Healer, Mind As Slayer*, 10
Perception, higher sense, 131–132
Pert, Candace, research by, 68–69
Philosophical orientations, 199–200
Playing detective technique, 139
Pleasant memory technique, 75
Psyche, Carl Jung on, 46
Psychoneuroimmunology (PNI), 65–66
  research, 67–68

R

Reason, Carl Jung on, 48
Reframing, 127–128
Regression
  inner advisor and, 124–125
  with inner guide, 124–125
  past life, 130–131
Rehearsal, age progressions, 128–129
Relaxation, 64–65
  California Nurses Association on, 98
  response, 64–65
    deepening, 76–77
  tension/progressive, 74
The Relaxation Response, 67
Religious
  orientations, honoring, 199–200
  symbols, 46
Renaissance, use of hypnosis during, 41–42
Reprogramming, 174–175
Responsibility, described, 6
Rheumatoid arthritis, autoimmune imagery and, 137
Rituals
  healing, 204–206
  initiation, 49
Rituals of Healing, 204–206

Role modeling, 208
Rossman, Martin, Academy for Guided Imagery and, 54, 63

S

Sacred
  defined, 201–202
  space, creating, 118–119
Scientific Revolution, imagery and, 66
Secretary's Commission on Nursing Report, 203–204
Self
  awareness, barriers to, 7–8
  imaging parts of, 122–124
  re–evaluation, need for, 8–9
Selye, Hans, stress and, 66
Sensation, Jung's definition of, 45
Sense perception, higher, 131–132
Shadow, concept of, 48–49
Shames, Karilee Halo, interview with, 146–150
Siegel, Bernie, 10
Simonton, O. Carl, 12, 71
  oncology imagery and, 106–107
  research by, 69
Software replacement imagery, 176
Special place
  clinical applications of, 79
  finding one's, 77–79, 89–90
  practical applications of, 79
Spiritual
  alignment, 141
  growth, 129–130
  nursing care
    autoimmune imagery and, 137–138
    contacting physical/nonphysical guidance, 132–133
    creating healing teams and, 133–134
    general, 129–130
    healing circle, 130
    higher sense perception, 131–132
    impending death and, 136–137
    negative influence avoidance, 135–136
    past life regressions, 130–131
Storytelling, symbology in, 52
Stress, Hans Selye on, 66
Survival, long–term, Caryle Hirshberg on, 166
Symbology
  Carl Jung on, 46–47, 49
  Clarissa Pinkola Estes on, 52
Symptoms, dialogue with, 112, 114–115

T

Teamwork, 190–191

Tension/progressive relaxation, 74
Theory of animal magnetism, Franz Mesmer and, 41
Therapeutic imagery, defined, 33, 71
Therapy, introductory experience, 21–31
  analysis of, 32
  concepts concerning, 34–36
Think & Grow Rich, 15
Thinking
  addictive, imagery and, 103–104
  Jung's definition of, 45
Time
  imagery and, 95–96
    examples, 96–97

Trauma, re–evaluating past, 127–128

U
Unknown, fear of, 48–49

V
Virchow, cell theory and, 43
Visualization
  creative, 53–54
  defined, 32–33, 71

W
Whole–person nursing care, setting boundaries, 179–181, 183
Wounded healer archetype, 202